# On Fire

by

G. Stone Johnson

On Fire

Published by JM Publishing
by G. Stone Johnson
Editing by David Jeffers
Photography by Ray Riggs

Cover design by Vivek Panwar

Copyright © 2016 G. Stone Johnson

This is a work of non-fiction. Some names of people and places have been changed. Any reference to a real name of a place, address or person is fully unintentional and under no circumstances was made to cause harm, intentionally or not.

World rights reserved. No part of this publication may be stored in a retrieval system, transmitted, or reproduced in any way including but not limited to photocopy, photograph, scan, facsimile, magnetic, or other record, without prior agreement and written permission of the publisher.

For information about permissions to reproduce any part of this work, write to
Printed in the United States of America

*To my Lord and Savior Jesus Christ*

*For my wife, Wendy
my sons, James & Matthew
my grandsons, Camden, Luke,
Jay, Nathanael
my mother, Frances
my father, Edward
my sister, Kathy
my brother, Carl
my nephew, Joshua
in remembrance of Sam*

# Table of Contents

PROLOGUE - ON FIRE .................................................................... 1
CHAPTER 1 - DAY IN, DAY OUT .................................................... 3
CHAPTER 2 - MONKEY BUSINESS ................................................ 13
CHAPTER 3 - STRANGER THAN FICTION .................................... 19
CHAPTER 4 - TAKING CARE OF OUR OWN .................................. 25
CHAPTER 5 - DANGEROUS FORCES ............................................. 32
CHAPTER 6 - EVERYDAY JUNK .................................................... 37
CHAPTER 7 - ALL IN A DAY'S WORK ........................................... 46
CHAPTER 8 - TRAGEDY AND COMEDY ....................................... 56
CHAPTER 9 - DARK TIMES ........................................................... 60
CHAPTER 10 - LAUGHING KEEPS YOU SANE ............................. 66
CHAPTER 11 - SOME DAYS DUTY IS FULL OF DOODY .............. 78
CHAPTER 12 - GENERAL HOSPITAL; DETROIT STYLE .............. 85
CHAPTER 13 - MAN'S BEST FRIEND ............................................ 91
CHAPTER 14 - INSTINCT ............................................................... 103
CHAPTER 15 - FAMILY FEUDS ..................................................... 109
CHAPTER 16 - CLOSE ENCOUNTERS ........................................... 117
CHAPTER 17 - FRICTION ............................................................... 127
CHAPTER 18 - DOGS ...................................................................... 133
CHAPTER 19 - MATTERS OF THE HEART ................................... 140
CHAPTER 20 - THE POWER OF HORSES ...................................... 150
CHAPTER 21 - HEROICS; FIGHTING FIRES AND SAVING CATS ............... 157
CHAPTER 22 - A GOOD DAY AT THE OFFICE ............................. 164
CHAPTER 23 - SOMETIMES YOU KICK, SOMETIMES YOU GET KICKED .. 176
CHAPTER 24 - WINTER WONDERLAND ...................................... 183
CHAPTER 25 - THEIR OWN WORST ENEMY ............................... 193
CHAPTER 26 - ON THE RUN .......................................................... 203

| | |
|---|---|
| CHAPTER 27 - ENDINGS AND BEGINNINGS | 211 |
| RETIREMENT POEM | 221 |
| AFTERTHOUGHTS | 223 |
| DEDICATION AND ACKNOWLEDGEMENTS | 226 |
| PHOTOGRAPHS | 228 |
| GLOSSARY | 245 |

# Prologue - On Fire

Sweat dripped off my right eyebrow, down my cheek and into the corner of my mouth. My partner was pushing me from behind into the raging fire. This was one of the hot-test fires I had ever been in. I had a tight grip on the inch and a half fog nozzle as we crawled deeper into the three bedroom home. We could feel the flames licking all around us and hear the crackling and popping sounds as the house was being devoured. The smoke was so thick that through my mask I could not see my hand in front of my face. All we could see was the ominous orange-red glow of the fire in every direction. The forty pounds of equipment I was wearing (Self Contained Breathing Apparatus, breathing mask, fire turnout gear and various other equipment) was starting to tire me out.

Suddenly, I could no longer feel the presence of my partner behind me. I reached for him, but he was gone. I turned slightly to look back, only to see the deadly glow of the fire was now blocking my only escape route. There was orange above me, orange to the right and the left of me, behind me and even below me. The red-hot embers on the floor were starting to burn my knees through my rubber boots. I tried to get up off the floor a bit, but the superheated gases around my head instantly burned my ears. I could feel the skin starting to peel, so I dropped back down to my knees. They would just have to burn! I sprayed water all around, but it seemed to make little difference. The glow above made me wonder how long before the ceiling would collapse. The sponginess beneath my hands and knees told me there was a good chance the floor could cave in. For the first time since becoming a firefighter, I was starting to wonder if I would get out of this one. For a split second, I wondered if I'd see my family again. Then my training kicked in, and I refocused my efforts on vigorously spraying water in every direction.

Finally, the orange started to fade. The heat began to decrease, and even the thick smoke was thinning out. Across the room, I could now see my fellow firefighters putting out the dying embers of the blaze. At last, I could get up off my burned knees. As I staggered to my feet, I realized I was in a kitchen. There wasn't much left. Charred remains of the cabinets, and unrecognizable globs of plastic on the blackened counter top were all that remained of this family's kitchen. A burnt-out shell filled with black piles of smoky, smelly, worthless junk.

As I made my way out of the ruins, I could see that the rest of the house was in relatively good shape, apart from the smoke damage. The once white walls were now gray from the floor to about four feet up, becoming blacker closer to the ceiling. Because the temperature was much higher near the ceiling, the paint up there was cracked and bubbled.

As I walked out of the house, I noticed one more thing. I saw what must have been a wall-mounted telephone, about four feet off the ground. Now, it was just a hardened stream of melted plastic dripping down to the floor. The heat of the flames transforms even the most mundane household objects into useless charred remains. I turned and walked out. My fire was over.

# Chapter 1 - Day In, Day Out

When I emerged from the house, the Captain ordered me to report to the paramedics to be checked out. They took my vitals (blood pressure, pulse, respiration) and then bandaged my knees and ears. I was then ordered to be taken to the hospital ER. On the way there, the paramedics and I talked about the fire.
"That was a hot one, huh?" John commented.
"Yes, it was!" I answered. "I have never burnt my knees before. This should be a good case for bunker pants."
 "We should be getting them next week," John replied. We turned into the hospital driveway. Once we were inside, the ER doctor put Silvadene on my ears and knees and bandaged them up.
He finished with an energetic, "You can go back to work now!" "Thanks a lot!" I said sarcastically.
 When we arrived back at Station Four on Hiller and Greer, the Engine was already cleaned and the fire hose was packed. Getting the Engine back in service after a fire was my least favorite thing, so I was glad that it was done. I had been assigned to drive the Res- cue that day. The Rescue was a paramedic truck that was a bit larger than an ambulance. The department used it for medical runs, rescues and fires.
In some fire departments, assignments are the same each day. At ours, however, roles changed regularly.
 "Dinner is on," said Ray, the watchman of the day. We took turns being on watch and one of the duties was to cook the meals. The delicious smell of baked chicken greeted me as I sat down at the table.
 "Sorry I left you in the fire. I had to get out," said Mike sheepishly, as he sat down next to me. "I'm not as young as I used to be," he said. He was older than the rest of us, and out of shape. The heat of the fire had been too much for him.
 I assured him it was alright. Everything had worked out. I had just reached for the mashed potatoes when the station alert tones screamed. Everyone groaned and started to rise from the table.

The dispatcher announced, "Station Four you have a car verses truck PIA (personal injury accident) with injuries on Haggerty and Pontiac Trail. Time out, 1923."

We all scrambled out the door to the apparatus room where the EMS, Rescue Four and Engine Four vehicles were waiting. I grabbed my fire turn-out gear, put it in the back of the Rescue and went around to the driver's side. I got in and started the diesel as Jerry climbed into the passenger side. The engineer, driving Engine Four, flipped on the master switch of the control panels. Red and yellow emergency lights began to flash. Jerry turned on our lights as well, adding to the cacophony of lights flooding the apparatus room.

Engine Four pulled out of the apparatus room onto the driveway. I could hear the diesel engine growling and smell the fumes as I drove the Rescue out behind the big vehicle. The sirens wailed and the air horns bellowed as we followed the Engine on to Hiller Road. It was almost pitch dark outside now, our red and yellow lights reflecting back at us off the shiny, wet blacktop. Over the radio I heard the officer in Engine Four say, "Engine Four and Rescue Four responding."

"Message received. Engine Four and Rescue Four responding," repeated the female dispatcher. As we gained speed, the adrenaline shot through my veins.

"I hope it's nothing serious," said Jerry. "I would like to be able to eat some time tonight!"

"That would be nice," I agreed. The apprehension I was feeling didn't really have to do with my waiting dinner. I just don't like car accidents. As we raced down Pontiac Trail, heading west towards the accident on Haggerty, a male dispatcher called, "Engine Four, Res- cue Four, police are on the scene. They report very serious injuries and would like you to step it up."

"Message received, dispatch," Jerry answered.

"So much for dinner," we both said at the same time.

We really could not "step it up" because the traffic was starting to back up. Soon it came to a dead stop. We pulled the Engine and the Rescue around the stopped traffic into the on-coming lane. Most of the cars pulled off the road so we could get through.

"There it is!" I called out.

"It's a bad one all right," said Jerry. As we pulled up closer, I could see the blue flashing lights of the three police cars parked around the scene. I pulled the Rescue up as close as possible. The Engine drove past to the other side of the accident in order to stretch an inch and a half line, just in case of a fire. As we came to a stop, I could see what looked like the frame of a car; just a frame. The rest of the mangled car body had been thrown about fifty yards down Haggerty Road.

It looked as though something had ripped the car's body off the chassis, crumpled it up into a ball and tossed it away like an unwanted toy. About twenty-five yards further on was a large, gray recycled-oil tanker, lying on its side in a field. As we got out of the Rescue, I saw three people in the car, still buckled into their seats, which were still securely fixed to the car's frame.

We moved closer to the eerie scene and saw that the seats were broken, lying back flat, with the passengers still buckled in tightly. When we got up to the vehicle, we discovered that they were all teenagers. The two in the front were girls. The one in the back was a boy. All of them looked lifeless. I went to the closest one, the boy. Jerry went to the two girls. I knelt over my patient. He had agonal respiration. I yelled to Jerry, "This one is trying to breathe!"

Jerry's quivering voice called back, "I don't think these two will make it." I glanced at the two girls as I reached to take the airway kit and LIFEPAK from Mike.

The girl who had been driving had brain matter coming out of her ears. The other girl had a severely broken neck and a depressed skull fracture. Neither was breathing. I heard the dispatcher announce that Rescue One was on its way.

I put down the equipment and felt for a pulse on the boy. There was none. Mike and I unbuckled his seat belt and laid him on a long wooden backboard on the ground. Using the air bag mask, I started to breath for him while Mike did chest compressions. As we performed CPR, I got a whiff of the old familiar stench that I've smelled so many times before in my career; a fatal combination of breath alcohol, dripping gasoline and blood.

Meanwhile, Jerry had the LIFEPAK and was checking for vital signs from the two girls. There were none. Jerry, realizing that there was no chance for the girls, came over to help me. He hooked up the LIFEPAK ECG to the boy and saw he was in ventricular-tachycardia. His ventricular heart rate was too fast to push any blood through his body. There wasn't a scratch on him, but he must have sustained massive internal injuries to be in this condition.

By this time, the second squad had arrived at the recycled-oil tanker. Bob, from the Engine Four crew, came over to help. He took over respirations so I could start an IV. I opened the IV kit, ripped the caps off the tubing and the bag of Ringer's lactate solution, and shoved the tubing into the bag.

At the same time, Jerry prepared to defibrillate the patient. He pulled the paddles out of the LIFEPAK, shouting, "Charging to 200 Joules!" Setting the dial to 200, he pushed the charge button on the side of the paddles. The LIFEPAK gave a high-pitched whine. When the sound stopped, we knew it was fully charged.

I grabbed scissors from the bag and cut off the boy's shirt. I then laid a gel pack on the right side of his chest and one on the ribs under his left arm pit. Jerry placed one paddle on each gel pack and yelled, "Clear!"

Everyone stepped back as Jerry pushed both buttons at the same time, discharging the electrical shock through the patient's chest, making his body jump. The ECG showed no change; still ventricular tachycardia and no pulse.

"Charging to 300 Joules!" Jerry said, as he changed the dial on the pack. Again, it whined as it charged. "Clear!" Jerry shouted, as he replaced the paddles on the patient's chest and defibrillated him for the second time. The patient lurched again, but still no change.

"Charging to 360 Joules!" This was the maximum charge a defibrillator could deliver. Jerry sent the pulse through the patient one last time, but there was no change.

"Resume CPR," I said with a sigh. We began to realize that this young teen probably would not make it. I picked up the IV bag of Ringer's, then opened the valve as the fluid made its way through the tubing, dripping onto the ground. I opened an 18 gauge needle, and someone handed me a tourniquet. I wrapped the elastic tightly around his upper arm, found a vein and stuck the needle in until blood started to seep out. I then shoved the tubing into the back end of the catheter and opened the IV wide. The fluids streamed into the patient's body. I removed the tourniquet and taped down the needle and tubing.

"Jerry, call St. Andrews Hospital for medical direction while I intubate the patient," I said. He nodded and left. I pulled the endo- tracheal tube and the laryngoscope out of the airway kit. Kneeling down in the mud over the patient's head, I opened his mouth. In my left hand I had the laryngoscope, and in my right hand I had an endo- tracheal tube. As I unfolded the L-shaped laryngoscope, the blade clicked down into place as the light snapped on. I gently slid the blade with the lighted end into the patient's mouth. I looked in and pushed it deeper until I could see his epiglottis. I put a little pressure in the blade and the epiglottis opened, exposing the larynx.

"I see the vocal chords," I said, carefully sliding the endotracheal tube between the two cyanotic vocal chords.

"It's in," I said with relief. The purpose of intubating an unconscious person is to get the best airway, and so that no stomach contents can be aspirated. Mike hooked the bag mask to the endotracheal tube sticking out of the patient's mouth and inflated the lungs. I picked up a stethoscope and held it to the patient's chest, making sure the tube was in the trachea and not the stomach.

Although I already knew it was in the right place, we had to double check. Mike squeezed the bag mask as I listened for the breath sounds.

"Good," I said, moving the stethoscope to the other side of his chest. Mike squeezed the bag again and I said, "This side is good too." I securely taped the tube in place as Jerry finished talking to the hospital.

"Dr. Jones wants one mg. of epinephrine." In response, I took out a preloaded 10cc syringe of epinephrine, popped off the caps, pushed all the excess air out and stuck the needle into the IV tubing. I depressed the plunger, emptying the contents into the patient's vein. No response. I tried another amp of epinephrine, but again no result.

"Dr. Jones wants us to start a dopamine drip and transport," Jerry reported. Jerry injected one gram of dopamine into a 500cc bag of dextrose and water, added an IV tubing and needle, then piggybacked it to the Ringer's tubing, letting the medication run at the proper drip rate into the patient.

"Let's get going," one of us said. We picked up the patient, now covered with tubes, mud and blood, on the backboard and placed him on the ambulance stretcher that had just arrived. We picked up the stretcher and rolled it into the back of the waiting ambulance. I jumped in to accompany my patient to the hospital.

Before I closed the door, I took in the accident scene. The flashing red, yellow and blue lights were pulsating and reflecting from all directions and surfaces. There were police cars, Rescues, fire Engines and firefighter gear everywhere. I got one more whiff of that horrible blood, gas and booze smell. I saw that the Rescue One crew was pulling the driver out of the overturned tanker up through the driver's side door. I pulled my head in and closed the door.

The ambulance had its emergency lights on as we turned onto Pontiac Trail. The police had cleared a path through traffic so we could get out. We sped towards the hospital. Even with lights and sirens and relatively little traffic, it seemed to take forever to arrive. There wasn't much left to do, except continue CPR, which the two ambulance crew members did. I gave some more epinephrine and defibrillated the patient again. The ECG changed to a normal sinus rhythm.

"Stop CPR!" I cried excitedly. I felt the teenager's carotid artery for a pulse. I looked for about eight seconds. "No pulse," I muttered with disappointment.

The ambulance attendant said, "Pupils are fixed and dilated. Are you sure there's no pulse? How could that be?"

"Resume CPR," I said, and went on to explain. "The electrical system of the heart is working, but the cardiac muscle has given up. There is just no blood left to push."

When we finally reached the hospital we were met by what seemed like a dozen doctors, nurses and orderlies. We wheeled the patient into the trauma room, and all of the doctors and nurses were shouting questions at the same time.

"What happened?"

"What kind of impact was it?"

"How long has he been without a pulse?"

"What's his name?"

"What history does he have?" "How old is he?"

"Where are his parents?"

The questions flooded over me. I tried to answer the best I could, but I had very little information to give them. All we had was the wallet in his back pocket. When we reached the trauma room, the medical personnel gathered around the young teen. They removed his clothes and examined him from head to foot. They patched him to their equipment. The hospital ECG now showed flat line, a-sys- tole, cardiac stand still. Dr. Jones stuck a long-needled syringe in his abdomen and drew out a barrel full of blood.

"All of his blood is in his abdomen," he announced. Dr. Jones took a scalpel and opened the teen's abdomen, exposing his intestines and other organs as blood squirted out. The doctor put his gloved hands into the abdominal cavity, searching for the injury.

"He has a lacerated liver, ruptured spleen and a torn inferior vein cava. That's it, nothing more we can do," declared Dr. Jones. "Time of death 2256."

All of the nurses and doctors started to walk away as they took off their surgical masks and ripped off their rubber gloves with a snap. A nurse came up to me.

"That was a bad one," she offered sympathetically. I replied,

"Yes it was and there are two more kids back at the accident scene."

Despite the emotional nature of these kinds of runs, you had to be able to maintain professionalism. I had to put aside the thought of those kids and get the paperwork done while the details were still fresh in my mind.

It took me about an hour to complete the medical report. I had to get it as accurate as possible, knowing I would probably have to testify in court sometime in the future.

During this time, the police officer who had been at the scene of the accident came into the hospital. From him I learned the preliminary information gathered. It was reported that the teens had run a red light, and the tanker driver tried to avoid colliding with the car, but ended up rolling over it instead. What a shame.

I finally got back to the station at about 0030. The place was quiet and dark. Everyone was sleeping. My dinner was wrapped and put away in the refrigerator, but I no longer had an appetite. I made my way across the kitchen to the dorm room door. It opened with a squeak as I tiptoed into the pitch black room. Fatigue took its toll as I reached my bunk. I took off my shoes, shirt and pants, but laid them out so I could get them on quickly if we got another run. I crawled into bed and tried to sleep.

As I began to drift off, the most horrible sound in the world penetrated my slumber; loud snoring from the other side of the dark room. Sleeping firefighters! I remember thinking, "How am I going to get to sleep with that noise?" It sounded like the Three Stooges snoring. Somehow, I fell asleep anyway. I was soon startled awake by the station tones. The lights in the bunk room flashed on, and everyone sat up. "Station Four, you have a possible suicide at 2332 Old Court Trail," the dispatcher announced.

The two other paramedics and I scrambled to get dressed while the remaining firefighters lay back down. We hurried to the watch room and looked up the street on the big wall map while Jerry found the address in the section map. We rapidly calculated the quickest route, then hopped into the

Rescue. This, of course, was before every phone had a built-in GPS map system. The apparatus room door opened, and we were on our way.

"Rescue Four enroute," said Jerry with his mouth against the mic.

"Rescue Four enroute," repeated the dispatcher. No one said anything on the way to the residence. We turned right onto Old Court Trail. A blue flash in the side mirror caught my eye. It was a police car pulling up behind us. I slowed so he could pass.

The dispatcher called again, "Rescue Four, stage in front of the house. Don't go in until the police secure the scene."

"Message received. Staging in front of the house," Jerry answered. Not long after we stopped, a police officer came walking up to the Rescue.

"Good morning!" the officer said. "Nice night for a suicide. He did quite a number on himself. He's in his office, just inside the door." He helped us carry the equipment into the house.

"He's in here." The police officer opened the dark, wooden door to the office. We entered the room and found a well-dressed, approximately 45 year-old male leaning back in his office chair. His feet were up on a large, shiny black expensive-looking oak desk. The desk was very neat with small stacks of official-looking papers in nice rows on either side of a set of gold ink pens. Next to these were his nicely polished brown shoes. He looked like he had just leaned back to relax; only he was obviously dead.

His face was ashen gray, and his eyes were wide open. In the corner of his mouth was a string of blood dripping to his shoulder. His hands were on his chest, clutching something. It was a 12-inch long pearl-handled dagger. It looked as though he had taken the dagger with both hands and slowly pushed the cold steel blade through his chest wall and his heart. The sharp tip of the blade protruded out of his back, with blood dripping onto the chair then down to the wooden floor, forming a puddle. He was still clutching the handle of the dagger.

Surprisingly, there wasn't much blood on his chest, except for the small red stain on his white dress shirt where the dagger had impaled him.

"Try to touch as little as possible, ok?" the police officer directed. "Ok," I said, "but we will have to send an ECG to the hospital." We placed the ECG pads on the dead man's chest. As we expected, the monitor showed a flat line. Jerry called the hospital as I hooked the LIFEPAK to the radio and transmitted the results to them. The doctor announced the time of death as 0322. The police officer entered the room as I removed the ECG pads.

"How is his wife doing?" I asked.

"She said she found him when she came home from a night out with the girls. She doesn't seem too broken up about it. I think they may both have been having an affair," the officer summarized. We turned the body over to the police officer, who would then call the medical examiner.

We walked out to the Rescue. As we were putting the equipment back into the truck, Jerry said to me, "What-a-way-to-go!" "Yeah," I replied. "That's how a real man would do himself." It was 0355 by the time we got back to bed. I was asleep when my head hit the pillow. Mercifully, no other runs came in that night. However, 7:30 a.m. still came very early.

I awoke to the smell of freshly brewed coffee and the clanging of pans in the kitchen. The watchman was emptying the dishwasher. I slowly got up and dressed, put my bedding away in my locker, and came out to the kitchen for a nice warm cup of joe.

All of the fire persons (we had one woman at Station Four) were sitting around the large dinner table sipping their coffee and dis- cussing the runs of the past shift. The Unit Two crew was starting to wander in. Rusty-Ray entered the station, his blond hair and stocky frame a familiar and welcome sight. Rusty was my best friend from when we were about three years old, and he now worked with me at the fire department. We used to do things together fairly often, but when he got hired he was put on Unit Two. After that, we hardly ever saw each other.

"Hi Rusty-Ray! How's the wife and kids?" I called him Rusty-Ray because his family and I had called him Rusty since we were kids, but everyone else calls him Ray.

"Everyone is great, Gregory," he stated. He was one of the few who called me by my full name.

"Rusty-Ray, my best buddy in the whole world!" I declared grandly.

"What do you need, Gregory?" Rusty asked, recognizing my "I-need-a-favor" tone.

"Could you cover me for the last half hour?" I pleaded.

"Sure, Gregory. No problem," Rusty agreed.

"Thanks, Rusty-Ray. We had a rough night," I explained, "and I'd like to go home and get some sleep."

"Go have a good sleep," said Rusty.

"Thanks. See you in the morning," I said. As I walked over to the sink to pour out my cup of joe, the station tones went off. Everyone jumped up from the table and hurried towards the watch room,
except for me. Rusty gave me a knowing look as he took my spot on the Rescue.

"Engine Four, Rescue Four, and Engine Three you have a structure fire at 4004 Draper Street!"

I watched the Engine and Rescue, with emergency lights flashing, pull out of the bay door. As they turned onto Greer Road, I saw Rusty-Ray shaking his fist at me. I chuckled to myself and closed the apparatus room doors.

Now it was quiet except for the TV that had been left on. I walked over and turned it off. I grabbed my fire gear and hung it up on the wall in the apparatus room with the rest of the off-duty fire gear. I slowly walked towards the exit, enjoying the silence. As I opened the door and stepped outside to the parking lot, I heard, "Engine Four, Rescue Four on the scene. Heavy smoke showing…"

The door slammed shut.

# Chapter 2 - Monkey Business

Getting home was my favorite part of the day, seeing the smiling faces of my family after working for twenty-four hours straight. I stepped through the door, anticipating being tackled by my eighteen-month old boy, Jimmy, and kissed by my lovely wife, Wendy. My smile turned into a slight frown. No one was there; no one except Ninja, my little seven-pound black dog.

"Where is every one, Ninja?" She just licked my hand in response, and I gave her a pat on the top of her head. Ninja looked like a Dr. Seuss character, with skinny long legs that didn't match the rest of her.

"How's Mugsy?" I asked, going up to the basket where my ancient dog slept. There was a lot of snoring coming out of that dog. I touched his head and he jumped.

"Did I scare you, Mugsy?"

He looked up at me with his milky-colored eyes, wagging his tail in recognition. He used to be a good watch dog, but now, at seven- teen-years old, his hearing and sight weren't what they used to be.

"Do you want to go outside?" I yelled in his ear. Mugsy just laid his head back down in his bed and resumed snoring.

"I guess not," I laughed.

Later that morning, I let Mugsy out to relieve himself. He started running around. That dog couldn't see or hear, but he sure could run, not that he could see where he was going. I called to him, like that would do any good. Poor Mugsy was bumping into things, and then he started running towards the pond behind the house.

The pond was about fifty feet wide, two hundred feet long and around fifteen feet deep. Mugsy barreled into the pond with me running after him. He started swimming. I called to him, but he couldn't hear. He swam blindly out towards the middle. If I didn't get him quickly, he would get too far away. Seeing no other choice, I jumped into the cold water after him and pulled him back to shore.

I had to take the dripping wet dog to the hose to rinse him off, then to the garage to dry him off with some towels. I led Mugsy back into the house and gave him a pat on the head.

"That was fun," I commented to my deaf dog. He panted happily and wagged his tail. The things we do for our pets, I thought to myself.

As I stood up, I noticed a stack of tissues sitting on the counter next to the tissue box. On the end table I spotted another stack of tissue, also neatly piled next to a tissue box. Both of the boxes had been completely emptied of their contents.

That seemed strange, so I looked around the house to see if the other tissue boxes were the same way. Sure enough, in the bathroom I found a third box in the same condition. This definitely seemed like monkey business to me. Walking back into the kitchen I found a banana and a peach with small bites in them.

"Beebe!" I yelled. "Where are you?" Beebe was a twenty year-old squirrel monkey that my dad had bought when I lived at home years ago. Beebe was back in his cage now, crouched snugly on his light bulb.

He must have gotten out of his cage somehow and played with the tissue boxes. I could understand why it intrigued him. In my mind, I could see how it must have happened. Beebe pulled out a tissue, but it was magically still there, so he set it down and pulled out another. There was still a tissue there! He probably kept it up until
he got bored. He left three piles of tissue on the table. Then he took a bite out of some fruit and returned to his cage, where he felt warm and safe.

I put some grapes and frozen peas in Beebe's cage and this time latched the door. The animals kept me as busy as the fire department did.

Usually my days off were filled with other obligations. Once I had five years on the job, I wanted to start my own business in my spare time. I didn't know what I wanted to do, but then an opportunity fell into my lap.

It just so happened that my father, Ed, was retiring from forty-four years of performing marionette shows. My father had been on TV in the 1950's, on a show called "Let Willy Do It." The show featured two of my father's marionettes: Applesauce the Dragon and Gee-Whizzer the Gremlin. Now, I was recovering Johnson Marionettes.

Dad didn't think I would be able to do it. I had to build a new stage and buy back a few shows that he had already sold. It was actually a perfect business for someone working in the Fire Department. I knew what my schedule would be a year in advance, and I consistently had days off during the week. Since my target audience was elementary schools, this worked out well.

On one rare day when my schedule was free and clear, I was enjoying my time off when the phone rang. It was Rusty. "Hey, Rusty. What can I do ya for?" I greeted him. "Can you work for me today?" he asked.

"Sure," I said. "When?"

"How about now? I have a practice for the Orchestra." "All right. I'll come in," I agreed.

Rusty was a multi-talented guy. Not only was he a firefighter, he was good at photography and was a professional percussionist with the Detroit Symphony Orchestra. They would occasionally ask him to sit in for another musician.

At WBFD (West Bloomfield Fire Department), we could trade blocks of time like Rusty and I were doing now. We could even trade whole days. We worked twenty-four hour shifts followed by twenty-four hours off. After our second shift in a week, we'd get three days off in a row.

Soon, I was in my car and pulling out of the garage. The area surrounding my house was heavily wooded and full of wildlife. I always had to pay attention. On this occasion, as I turned left out of my subdivision heading toward Station Four, I had to slam on my brakes to avoid three deer crossing the road. There was a big doe and two smaller ones that must have just lost their spots. Once they cleared the road, I started to push on the gas.

Suddenly, a huge eight-point buck bounded out of the tree line after the does. I watched him run across Commerce Road and disappear into the woods. Deer are a frequent road hazard in suburban southeast Michigan, causing plenty of accidents and more work for us.

As I walked into the living area at Station Four, I caught sight of Rusty. He smiled at me in greeting and said, "Thanks for coming in. It's been quiet all day, so maybe you'll get lucky." Just as he finished saying that, the tones for a run went off.

"Station Three and Station Four, you have a car versus tree PIA on Commerce Road west of Keith Road. Time out, 0934," the dispatcher announced. "You're driving the Rescue," said Rusty-Ray with a sheepish grin while I grabbed my gear. I jumped in the driver's side. Kenny, who was short and had a rather large stomach, jumped into the passenger side. Dave, a young, tall skinny guy, rode in back.

"Rescue Four responding," Kenny announced into the mic. "Engine Three responding," said a voice from the radio. We pulled out of the Station Four apparatus room as Kenny flipped on the red switch for the siren on the dashboard. The siren screamed, sending cars on both sides of the road off onto the shoulders.

As we pulled onto Hiller Road, one driver would not get out of the way. Kenny pushed the air horn with a loud blast. The car still would not yield the right of way. Looking around the car ahead, we saw that all the other cars were pulled off the road. I was able to pull around the uncooperative vehicle by using the oncoming lane.

As we approached the intersection of Hiller and Commerce Road, the light turned red. Kenny turned the siren to high/low and honked the air horn. I had to slow the Rescue, looking each way to make sure there were no vehicles approaching. It was clear, so we continued through the intersection, turning right onto Commerce Road.

All the vehicles in front of us were stopped on the side of the road, except for one blue car coming towards us in the oncoming lane. The driver of the blue sedan panicked and pulled into our lane, coming straight at us. I jerked the steering wheel to the right, swerving onto the dirt shoulder, just missing the car.

"Crazy drivers," Kenny said after taking a deep breath.

We were almost there when we heard, "Engine Three is on the scene." About a minute later, Engine Three came into view, its red lights flashing. It was parked on the right side of the road. We looked around, but didn't see an accident.

"Where is the car?" Kenny asked.

Then he announced on the mic, "Rescue Four on the scene." We looked around the area, and then I spotted it.

"There it is," I said, pointing up. And there it was; a Corvette…stuck up in a tree.

I parked the Rescue behind Engine Three. We got out of the truck and walked under the beautiful shiny red car, suspended ten feet above us. The tree was approximately fifteen to twenty feet tall, with a thick trunk and a bushy canopy. It stood in a large grassy field, with no other trees within three hundred yards in any direction.

An extension ladder was removed from Engine Three by its crew on my left. The driver of the Corvette, still in the tree, was trying to figure out how to get out of his car. "Get me down!" he finally yelled.

"Stay put! We will get you down!" I called back.

First, we made sure that the vehicle was secure in the branches. Then we raised the extension ladder up to the car. One firefighter from Engine Three butted the ladder, putting his feet on the base, his hands a few rungs up, leaning on it for stability. We never got on a ladder without one or two firefighters butting it.

I climbed up to the car and asked the driver "Are you hurt?" "No, not yet," the guy replied. "Not until I get home."

He had gray hair, with a beer belly and a large red nose. I noticed he was wearing a large gold chain around his neck, a gold bracelet on his right wrist and a golden Rolex on his left wrist.

"Are you sure you're not hurt?" I repeated.

"No, I'm not hurt," the driver assured me.

"Ok, let me help you down the ladder," I said. Sticking my head through the open car window, I immediately detected a mix of new car smell and the alcohol on the driver's breath. The stench hit me like a punch in the nose.

"How did you get your car up here?" I asked the drunk driver. Technically, we were not allowed to say that someone was drunk until he had been tested, but this was an obvious case.

"I don't know," he said, with a smelly smirk. I carefully helped him out of his seat and down the ladder. Once on the ground, we walked him to the Rescue and checked him out more carefully. He did not have a scratch on him, and his vitals were normal, but his breath reeked of alcohol.

The police officer poked his head into the back of the Rescue and asked, "Is he ok to take a Breathalyzer?"

"He's good to go," I said.

"Sir, have you had anything to drink recently?" the officer asked.

"Just a few drinks," the driver replied reluctantly.

The officer walked the guy to his squad car, put him into the back seat and closed the door. Turning to my partner, I asked, "How did the Corvette get up there?"

He said, "The officer told me he was going about 90 mph when he became airborne. How he became airborne we may never know."

Shaking our heads, we walked towards the Rescue. Suddenly, we heard the fire tones going off again. "Station One and Station Four, you have a PIA on Orchard Lake Road, south of Maple."

As we hopped in the Rescue, over the radio we heard, "Rescue One is out-of-service."

"This is Rescue Four," Kenny announced. "Message received. Rescue Four responding."

Some days, the monkey business had no end.

# Chapter 3 - Stranger Than Fiction

We did a U-turn onto Commerce Road as Kenny flipped on the lights and siren. This time all the cars were compliant, pulling over to the side of the road as we accelerated back towards Hiller.

"Engine Two is responding," said a voice over the air.

As we entered the intersection, the dispatcher said, "Rescue Four, be advised: police are on the scene and report only one car involved with three injuries."

"Message received," Kenny responded.

We turned north onto Old Orchard Trail, a narrow ribbon of pavement that wound around Orchard Lake. There was no shoulder on the Trail, meaning drivers had nowhere to go to let us pass safely. As we made our way around the lake, a big brown UPS truck suddenly stopped in front of us.

I had to slam on the brakes and swerve into the oncoming lane to avoid crashing into the truck. Good thing I had already noticed that there were no vehicles coming toward us. Having driven on this road many times, I knew that you always look far ahead to make sure no vehicle is in the way. I swerved back into our lane once I passed the truck.

Ahead of us, I could see that all the cars were stopped, but still on the road. I had to swerve in and out of our lane around the cars, like a slalom skier, until we reached Pontiac Trail.

As we turned left, we heard, "Engine One on the scene." When we reached the intersection of Pontiac Trail and Orchard Lake Road, the traffic light was red. I slowed down to wait for the traffic to clear, but the cars would not stop. Kenny pushed the air horn with a loud "hooooonk!" The cars kept on coming.

You can't just enter an intersection, even with lights and sirens going. Cars will still hit you. The purpose of the sirens and lights is to ask for the right of way, not to permit you to blow a red light. Finally, the cars stopped and we slowly proceeded through the intersection and turned right onto Orchard Lake Road.

Over the radio, we heard "Rescue Four, be advised: the police report serious injuries. Better step it up!" Kenny answered, "Message received."

I said to Kenny, "I hate it when they say that. Don't they know we are going as fast as we can?" We accelerated to about 60 mph, sirens wailing as we passed first Walnut Lake Road and then Maple Road.

As the accident scene came into view, I could see the emergency lights flashing on all the vehicles. A small pickup truck, with a police car in front and one in back, was at center stage. Engine Two was parked beside the pickup, blocking the lane. Two police officers directed traffic.

I slowed the Rescue, noticing a small flatbed trailer with rails around it. It faced us with its tongue dug into the pavement. I didn't give it much thought as we arrived at the accident site.

Kenny reached for the mic, calling "Rescue Four on the scene."

"Message received, Rescue Four," answered the dispatcher. I pulled the vehicle up behind the Engine. As we got out, Jerry, the lieutenant from Engine One, met us at the door.

In a serious tone he gave us an update "There are three injuries and one possible K, but we don't know what caused the accident yet." Kenny and I exchanged a glance. K is shorthand for "killed." This wasn't going to be pretty.

We walked to the pickup truck and found that two of the three victims were out of the truck and talking to police. The third person was still sitting in the vehicle.

I motioned to Dave, who was carrying the medical boxes, "You take the two with the police." He nodded and went on his way. Kenny and I looked in the truck. In the passenger seat was a man in his forties. He was obviously dead, his face grayish white.

I noticed that his head was leaning back on the head rest. He had shoulder length hair and a goatee. His mouth was partly open, and his pupils were dilated. Reaching through the open car door, I checked his neck for a pulse.

"No pulse," I quietly said. I observed that he had a tear in his side, under his ribs. It was about the size of his fist, and blood dripped down from it between the seat and the door. His abdomen was slashed wide open, and his intestines had spilled onto his lap. They looked unreal, like they were made of colorless semi-transparent wax. There was no blood at all from that wound, but the smell was terrible. The best way to describe it is if you had field dressed a deer but mixed everything with gasoline. Not pleasant.

A police officer came up behind us and asked, "What's the patient's status?"

"He's gone," Kenny answered.

"Should I call the ME?" the officer asked.

"Yes, call the Medical Examiner. There is nothing we can do for him," Kenny replied. Dave walked up to where we were standing.

"The other two didn't have a scratch! So what killed him?" the police officer asked incredulously. We were trying to figure that out, as well.

I looked at the surreal sight in the truck, and noticed a perfect round ball of what looked like fat right beside the body. It was wax colored with just a tinge of blood. "Look at that," I said to the guys, pointing at the ball.

"I wonder what that's from?" Kenny asked. We looked around, trying to understand what had caused this bizarre injury. Meanwhile, Dave slapped the ECG on the body as protocol dictated. As we expected, he got a flat line. Kenny volunteered to call the hospital.

We have to call the hospital, even when the victim has expired, so a doctor can officially pronounce him dead. Kenny went to the other side of the truck and used the radio in the big duffle bag to contact the hospital staff.

"Something went through the car door," Dave said, pointing to a hole. It was about the size of a fist and went all the way through the door. We could see blood on the inside of the hole.

"I wonder what made *that*?" I asked out loud. Then, I remembered the trailer from down the road. I signaled for Dave to follow me as I walked over to it. We examined it closely. Dave found blood on the tongue of the trailer. The pieces of this puzzle began falling into place.

"The trailer tongue must have punctured the truck door and went through his side, opening up his abdomen. See that hollow part of the tongue? The one that holds the ball of the trailer hitch? When it came back out, it must have carved out the ball of fat like an ice cream scoop and it fell onto the seat," I surmised. When Kenny joined us, we told him our theory. He suggested we let the police officers know what we had discovered.

As we walked back up to the accident scene, a large pickup pulled in beside one of the police cars. The driver got out to talk to the officer. A few minutes later, the officer put the guy into the back of the squad car.

When we returned to the accident site, the officer got out of his car and told us, "We have an ID on the victim. He was returning home from an Alcoholics Anonymous meeting at Henry Ford Hospital on Maple Road when this pickup," he gestured to the recently arrived vehicle, "hauling that trailer," he pointed at the trailer, "was passing by in the oncoming lane. The trailer broke free. The driver didn't even know he had lost the trailer until he got home. Then, when he came back to try to find it, he spotted the accident. So, he stopped to talk to us. He said he didn't have a safety chain on the trailer. I'll be taking him to jail."

The officer continued, "Earlier, witnesses said they saw the trailer come loose, traveling at about 60 mph towards the victim's pickup. The driver swerved to avoid the trailer, but it impacted the pickup anyway."

I told the officer our idea that the tongue of the trailer had impaled the passenger and disemboweled him.

"That makes sense," the officer said. "I guess he never knew what hit him."

"Man, this will be a lot of paper work," said Kenny. "It will most likely end up in court." About that time, the ME pulled up in a white van and was met by the police.

"I guess it's time to get back in service," I said, heading back to our vehicle. I grabbed the hand radio from my belt and said, "Rescue Four in service."

"In service received, Rescue Four," responded the dispatcher. To my surprise and delight, it was a quiet ride back to Station Four.

When we pulled into the station driveway Kenny called in, "Rescue Four at quarters."

"At quarters received, Rescue Four."

The large bay door opened, and I backed the truck into the stall. Rusty was waiting in the watch room and pushed the green button on the wall to close the apparatus room door.

"Hi Gregory!" called an overly cheerful Rusty-Ray. "Have a run while I was gone?"

"I was out the entire time," I replied, shooting daggers with my eyes. "You owe me," I said.

"So sorry," Rusty answered back. "Well, thanks for coming in for me."

"You're very welcome. I'll see you in the morning," I said, walking towards the door. Home sounded good right about then. As I pulled into the driveway at home, I noticed I was in the Rescue vehicle.

"How could I have gotten into the Rescue instead of my car?" I asked myself. "How could I be so stupid?" As these questions raced through my brain, I began to sweat, thinking of the consequences of this mistake.

I kept thinking, "I am going to get into so much trouble. Maybe I can get it back to the station before anyone notices, definitely before a run comes in."

Shaking and sweating profusely, I slammed the Rescue into reverse, my mind still churning. "They'd still be having morning coffee," I thought. "Maybe if I hurry, I can return the truck before they notice."

I put the Rescue into drive and stepped on the gas. Then I heard the familiar first two tones that meant WBFD had a run. My heart sank as I waited for the third tone that would indicate which station was to respond. I waited... and waited. The last tone went off.

"Station Four, you have...to get up. Honey, wake up!"

The alarm was from my clock radio. My beautiful wife was trying to wake me up. "Ok, I'm getting up," I protested. "I had that dream again," I said, trying to shake the cobwebs of sleep from my head.

"Which dream?" Wendy asked.

"The one where I'm driving the Rescue home by accident." She nodded in recognition. Wendy was no stranger to the life of a firefighter. Her dad, Bob, had been a volunteer at Station Three. On the day I met my wife, I was assigned to that station for the day. Bob and the other guys were playing cards, but I was done losing. So instead, I got my guitar, sat on a wooden chair and started to play some James Taylor.

A cream colored Cadillac drove up and parked outside the station. The most beautiful young lady I had ever seen got out of the car. She had dark hair and bright blue eyes. A few minutes later Bob introduced her to me, saying, "This is my daughter Wendy. Could you show her the new Rescue?"

"Of course," I agreed.

I showed Wendy the Rescue, and the next day we started dating. I know she was sent from God because only a confluence of unusual circumstances allowed us to meet in the first place. First, she had never been to the fire station before. Second, I was only at Station Three for the day. Finally, her father's truck had broken down and he
had called home for Wendy to bring him the part he needed. If any of those things hadn't occurred, we would have never met. I doubt Bob realized then that he would become my father-in-law soon after that. In the few years we had been married, Wendy was already accustomed to the dreams I'd have about the Department.

"I'm not surprised," Wendy told me. "You were so exhausted, you fell straight into bed. Now it's time to get up and do it all over again. It must feel like you never left."

"Yeah, definitely," I answered, throwing the blankets off and sitting up. I slowly settled down from the emotions the nightmare had stirred up.

A few minutes later, I swung my feet out of bed and headed to the bathroom to start getting ready.

I was in the shower when I heard the telephone ring. As I shut off the water, Wendy called to me. "Station One called. You have to go to Station Three today."

"Ok," I yelled back as I dried off. I quickly threw my uniform on. I pinned my badge on my light blue shirt.

"I'm late!" I grumbled, looking at the clock. "Wendy, will you please feed the monkey? Thank you," I added, giving her a kiss as I walked to the front door. A memory suddenly popped into my head. I turned to Wendy and asked, "Do you remember when you cooked me breakfast and burned the monkey?"

Wendy cringed, "Yes, I do. Poor Beebe."

I kissed her good bye again and walked to my car. As I drove to Station Three, I reflected on Beebe's misadventure. Just after Wendy and I were married, she wanted to surprise me with a nice breakfast when I got home from work. Beebe had gotten out of his cage and wanted to get up on the counter. Grabbing the cord of the coffee maker, he began to climb. The pot full of hot coffee poured down all over him.

Screaming, he ran down the basement stairs. Wendy tried to put cool water on him, but he would not get close to her. When I got home, Beebe would not come to me either. Needless to say, we ate a cold breakfast that day.

Beebe hid for several hours. Eventually, he came around and I took him to the vet, who applied Silvadene on his burns. He had almost died, but he did recover, eating and squealing once again. Beebe had scars and large patches of fur missing all over his little body. Burns are a horrible injury to have, even for a little monkey.

# Chapter 4 - Taking Care of Our Own

I pulled into the driveway at Station Three. The apparatus room door stood open, revealing fellow firefighter Bob's tall, stocky frame. He was waving frantically to me as if to say "get in here now!"

I parked my truck. Bob met me at my door saying, "I'm the only one here and we have a possible house fire! Go grab your gear. You'll drive."

Bob had come in early for someone and found himself alone with a call. I'm sure he was glad to see me arrive! I quickly threw on my gear and hopped into the driver's side of Engine Three. I started the vehicle, and the diesel fumes filled the apparatus room. Turning to Bob, I asked, "Where to?"

"Head to Station One's area; turn left," he answered. I released the air brake, pushed the clutch in and put the Engine into first gear. Bob set the map on the dashboard and stepped on the siren switch in the floor. The siren screamed as Bob flipped the lights on. I slowly released the clutch and pulled the Engine out onto the driveway. As I was getting ready to enter the road, Bob called out, "Clear to the right." Seeing that there was no traffic to my left, I pulled out onto Green Lake Road.

Engine Three was the only fire engine left in the township with a standard transmission. This meant I had to double clutch when shifting. Here's how it worked: I pushed in the clutch and revved the engine. I put the engine in neutral, let off the clutch, revved the engine, pushed the clutch back in, slipped the transmission into second gear and let up on the clutch one last time. Miraculously, the transmission did not grind, which is what usually happened when I shifted into second gear.

As we turned onto Commerce Road, I heard the radio call over the sound of the siren, saying "Engine One responding to the possible house fire."

The dispatcher responded, "Message received, Engine One." We turned right onto Old Orchard Trial, me struggling to double clutch the engine into third as we drove around Orchard Lake. I slowed as we approached the light at Pontiac Trail, double clutching back down to first gear. It was such a pain to drive!

As we headed towards Orchard Lake Road, we heard, "Engine One on the scene, reporting smoke showing on a three-story house. We will be pulling the cross-lays."

"Message received, Engine One," said the dispatcher. I pulled right onto Orchard Lake Road, drove past Station One, turned left on Maple Road and finally made a right onto Middle Belt Road. Bob was checking the map to see where the hydrants were located.

Over the air we heard, "Engine Three, we need you to stretch to the hydrant." We were carrying three-inch hose, used to hook up the Engine to the hydrants.

"Engine Three to Engine One, message received," Bob responded. Then, to me he said, "There is a fire hydrant to the east of the house."

"Ok, east of the house," I confirmed. We had gone about one hundred yards when I noticed a large set of skid marks on my side of the road. They led across the pavement and past the left shoulder.

Over the radio we heard, "Engine One is getting ready to enter the house."

"Engine One ready to enter the house, received," the dispatcher replied. My eyes followed the long skid marks across someone's yard right up to a large tree.

There was a police car smashed against it, smoke coming out from under the hood, blue lights still flashing. I slowed down to take a better look. "Bob!" I yelled, pointing to the accident. "A cop car crashed into a tree!" I slowed the Engine to a stop.

Bob protested, saying, "We have to get to the fire!" "But a police officer needs our help!" I pointed out.

Putting the Engine in park, I grabbed the orange first-aid kit and ran down the long tire tracks to the police car. An officer from WBPD was slumped over the steering wheel, unconscious. Blood streamed from his forehead, as he made a snoring sound. There was still white dust from the deployed air bag hanging in the air. I yelled to Bob, "He is badly injured! We need to get the Rescue here!"

"Are you sure we need a Rescue?" Bob asked.

"YES, we need the Rescue!" I yelled back, grabbing a bandage from the first aid kit. As I bound the officer's forehead, trying to control the bleeding, I noticed he was breathing all right. However, he was still snoring.

I could hear Bob call the dispatcher for a Rescue through my hand radio. The dispatcher answered, "All the Rescues are out at the hospital or at the fire."

Then we heard "Engine One to radio, fire is through the roof!" "Through the roof, Engine One," was repeated.

I got into the back seat of the police car and cradled the officer's head in my hands to put traction on his neck. I hoped he hadn't fractured it, but with the violence of this crash spinal injuries were a likely possibility.

Bob came over to the car. "What do you need?"

"I need you to take over the neck traction," I replied. Bob got next to me in the back seat and took over. Turning to me he said, "They are going to pull the Rescue crew from the fire. It'll be here in about five."

"Good," I nodded as I pulled the cervical collar out of the first aid box. I carefully placed it around the officer's neck. He was still making a snoring sound when he breathed.

I looked at the officer's face. I didn't recognize him, but I did recognize his name. The tag on his uniform said "Jones." He was someone I played softball with.

This was the first time that I'd ever worked on someone I knew personally. I used the blood pressure cuff from the orange box and took his vitals. His pressure was 110/60; a little low, but as long as it did not get any lower, it would be all right. We would have to watch it, though. His pulse was 120 BPM, a little fast. It could have been a sign of internal injuries, but I figured not in this case.

I checked Jones over for any other injuries, starting with his chest, because he may have injured it with the steering wheel. He had a bulky bulletproof vest under his blue shirt, which rose and lowered with each breath. I felt under his vest, but didn't feel any deformity.

I noticed his gun belt, patent black leather with hand cuffs attached and pepper spray secured. His gun, however, was dangling out of his holster. I decided that I would worry about that later. I checked his arms and legs next. Fortunately, I did not find any other obvious injuries.

Just then, the Rescue pulled down the driveway and stopped next to the squad car. I looked back at the officer and saw the gun teetering in his holster, about to fall out. As he inhaled, the gun dropped and I snatched it just before it hit the ground. I handed it over to another officer that had just arrived. Cooper was the name on his shirt. He was of average height and had reddish hair.

As Officer Cooper took the gun out of my hand, he said, "Nice catch. Thanks. How's he doing?"

I summarized the situation for him. "He is breathing ok, but he has a head injury. I don't know how extensive it is or if there are spinal injuries."

At that moment John and Steve, paramedics from Rescue One, were standing over me. "What do you have?" Steve asked.

"Officer Jones has a head injury from hitting the steering wheel," I reported. I told them his blood pressure and pulse, and that we had also put a cervical collar on him. Steve took Officer Cooper aside to get the medical history for Jones as best as he could.

Over the radio we heard, "Rescue One, Officer Jones' family has been notified, and they will be waiting at the hospital." "Message received, dispatch," Steve responded. "Ok," I said, "time to pack him up."

John had brought both a long and short backboard from the rear of the Rescue. "I'll take the short board," I said as I reached for the wooden board. Bob was still holding the injured officer's neck.

We would use a short backboard to get a patient with suspected back injuries out of a car. We use it like a splint, so as not to make the patient worse off than when we found him.

In movies and on TV, you see rescue workers yanking people out of cars moments before they explode. In 30 years of experience, I have never seen a car explode. Generally, if a vehicle is going to catch on fire it will do so on impact. Besides, unless a patient is in dire condition, we have time to do things the right way, making sure not to paralyze the injured person.

I told Bob, "Keep up the traction while we push him forward far enough to put the short backboard behind him."

I couldn't get the board in position, so I said, "Push him a little more forward." Bob did as I asked, and I finally maneuvered it behind Officer Jones. I had to make sure that the board was right on the seat behind him.
Once the board was in place I said, "Ok, let's strap him down." Steve had gone to the passenger side seat to help.

We took the lower strap on the left side and put it around and under the outside of his leg, up between his legs, fastening it to the top strap on the opposite side. We did the mirror image of this with the straps on the other side, making a crisscross pattern.

Bob strapped Jones' head down on the wooden board so he couldn't move it. These days, the boards are mostly made of plastic, but we mainly had wooden or metal ones. The officer was packaged and ready for us to extract him. I said to the other medics, "Let's lift him out head first, on three."

Steve was in the passenger seat. Bob was in the back seat, and I was beside Officer Jones outside the car. "One! Two! Three!" Steve lifted Jones' legs up as Bob picked him up by the straps. Simultaneously, I lifted his left side using the straps.

"Keep his legs up," I warned. We had to do this because the straps were tight and could cause further injury. We maneuvered Jones on to his side and started pulling him out head first.

"Is the long board ready?" I asked.

"Right behind you," John said. As we pulled Jones out, I felt the long board slide past me and rest on the car seat.

Together, we had pulled him most of the way out when John said, "Let me take the head." I moved, allowing John to take my position. I moved to the legs. Steve and Bob were out of the car now and helped lift Officer Jones onto the long board. We carried him a short distance to the stretcher that was waiting.

"Down on three. One, two, three!" John counted. Since John was at the officer's head, he was in charge of directing us to move the patient. We set Jones down on the stretcher, and I uncoupled the straps holding his legs up and slowly let them down. Once the patient was safely on the stretcher, we got him to the Rescue and into the back. I climbed in with him and started an IV. We rode to the hospital, where we were met by a doctor and nurse. We lifted the stretcher out of the Rescue and wheeled Officer Jones into the emergency room. We gave the doctor and nurse the report while they worked on him, and then they took over. Before leaving, I talked to Officer Jones' wife to reassure her as best I could.

I got in the Rescue with the others and headed back to the fire. By the time we got back, they were just rolling up the fire hose. The inch and a half and two and a half were already done, but the three inch hose still had to be put away.

The inch and a half and two and a half inch hoses are fifty feet long and made of cloth on the outside, rubber on the inside, coupled together with aluminum or brass. The three inch hose is one hundred feet long and made of yellow rubber. All the hose had to be uncoupled, rolled up and taken to the station to be washed, dried and put on the hose rack. Once it was dry, the hose would then be repacked on the Engine.

The three inch hose is the only one repacked on the Engine at the scene. Being filled with water and too heavy to carry, we had to uncouple it to let it

drain. Then we rolled it up, pushing the rest of the water out along the way, then repacking it back on Engine Three. The whole process, including the drive back to Station One, took about
an hour. We still weren't finished, though. Washing Engine One and repacking it took even more time. It's tiring but necessary work. Just as we finished, I saw a police car pull in to the station. An officer got out and walked into the Chief's office.

Bob turned to me and said, "It's time to get back." I nodded. "I'm ready."

"Johnson!" The Chief's voice caught my attention. I turned toward him as he called out, "In my office!"

"I'll be right in, Chief," I responded. I looked at Bob, who shrugged his shoulders. Neither one of us knew what this was about.

I went through the glass door between the apparatus room and the watch room to the Chief's office. I knocked.

"Come in," said the muffled voice behind the door. I entered the office. "Johnson," the Chief simply said in greeting.

"Chief?"

"You know Officer Miller?" He indicated the dark-haired man stood in front of his desk. Although this guy was about my height, the considerable bulk added by the early kind of body armor made him look somewhat like a mountain.

I nodded, saying, "We've been on a number of runs together."

Turning to the officer, I greeted him with, "Good to see you again."

"The pleasure is all mine," he replied, adding, "Officer Jones is a friend of mine. The Police Chief is at the hospital with him now."

"How is he doing?" I asked.

"He is still unconscious. He's had a CT scan which showed a possible brain injury. The doctors don't think its life threatening, but he will need therapy for quite some time." He paused a moment as I took this all in.

"Also the Chief and I would like to thank you for stopping instead of continuing to the house fire."

"Of course I stopped. We couldn't pass by one of West Bloomfield's finest in trouble," I answered.

"Well, the Chief wanted me to stop by and thank you," Officer Miller added.

"You're very welcome," I replied, adding, "keep us informed of Officer Jones' progress,"

"I will," Miller agreed. "And see you on the next run." He turned to the door and walked out.

Turning to me, the Chief said, "It's a good thing you stopped!" "Yeah, I guess!" I agreed. "But, really, what else could we do?" "Well, that's true" he paused. "Get back to Station Three," he added in dismissal.

"Ok, Chief. I'm out of here."

When Bob saw me he called out, "So, J?" Jay was what he liked to call me. "What did the Chief want?"

"He just wanted to tell me you suck," I joked.

Bob's big jaw loosened just a bit, letting a little smile spread his lips. "Talking about me behind my back again, eh?"

"Not me! It was the Chief!" I defended myself. "Chuck you, Farley," Bob said. "Let's go home."

# Chapter 5 - Dangerous Forces

After we returned. to the station, we decided to get subs for lunch. "How about Tubby's?" I asked Bob.
"Sounds good to me."
"I'll go get it," I offered.
Tubby's was popular with us because they would give firefighters half off. We always appreciated hearty food, and getting it cheaper was even better.
Once I returned with the sandwiches, we sat down to enjoy the meal. As we ate, I got a call from the officer at Station One. "Johnson, you are going to Station Four on your next day."
After hanging up the phone, I turned to Bob and asked, "Why can't I ever stay at the station that I am assigned to?"
Bob didn't have an answer, but I hadn't really expected one. I was used to being regularly transferred out to other stations because I had the seniority to be in charge. Since I was from the first group of five firefighters to have paramedic training in the entire department, I had seniority from early on in my career. I quickly got used to being moved to whichever the station needed me. It was part of the job.
The rest of the day had been quiet, but just as I was ready to hit the sack, the tones went off. Bob and I stood up from the table and walked to the watch desk in the other room. As we reached the watch room, the third tone told us it was for Station One. We breathed a sigh of relief. Not for us.
"You have a medical emergency at 2332 Woodrow Wilson, Time out, 2344," said the dispatcher.
Not being for us, we headed back to the living area. I turned on the TV, and we sat back down at the table. Bob got up to get some chips when the tones went off again.
"This time it has got to be for us," I told Bob. We got to the watch desk when the last tone was about to sound out. It seemed like a long pause before Station Four's tone went off.
"Station Four, you have a smoke investigation at 6640 Hiller Road." Still not for us.

We had just sat down again when the tones went off a third time. We heard four tones, which meant two stations would be going. The fourth tone was ours. "Rescue Two and Engine Three, you have a PIA across from 2314 Long Lake Road. Police are enroute. Time out, 0000 hours (midnight)."

From the watch desk, Bob keyed the mic and said, "Engine Three responding."

"Responding Engine Three at 0001," dispatch confirmed.

We hopped in the Engine. We didn't say much, because we both knew where we were going. This same stretch of road seemed to get a lot of accidents. I turned on the battery switch next to the seat and pushed the start button, bringing the diesel engine to life. I could smell the fumes as the door in front of us rose enough to let us out.

Bob turned on the headlights and the emergency lights as we pulled left on Green Lake Road. I could see the red lights reflecting off the wet road as we went forward. It was dark now and there was a slight drizzle coming down. When we were near the end of Old Orchard Trail, Rescue Two came on the air.

"Rescue Two has a flat tire and will be slow getting to the scene," said a voice over the radio.

"Engine Three," the dispatcher responded, "you will be there by yourself." About a minute later, we arrived near the scene.

"Engine Three in the area," Bob called in. A fog had settled over everything, making it difficult to see. Bob turned on the side spot light and pointed it in the direction where we thought the incident was. The beam of light reflected off the fog, but nothing else was visible. Through the mist a gray shape appeared in front of us. As it came into view, Bob called in the mic, "Engine Three on the scene."

We crept closer and Bob shouted, "What the heck is that?" He jotted down the time when the dispatcher called back.

"Engine Three on the scene 0005."

Bob set the paper down on the dash, knowing he'd need it for the report after we got back. I slowly pulled the Engine next to what looked like the back half of a large car. Bob shone the light ahead farther. There was the front half about one hundred feet ahead.

"It looks like a car ripped in half!" Bob yelled.

I stopped the Engine and put on the parking brake, turning on the side lights before stepping out of the vehicle. The back half of the car was pointing away from us. We could see the tail lights. We walked around to the front of it.

The sharp, jagged edges of the torn metal grabbed my bunker pants and stopped me. I had to back up to get unhooked. Bob said with a grin, "Watch out for the sharp edges."

"Thanks, Bob," I replied with equal sarcasm. "Empty. No one here," Bob said.

The only thing in the back seat was a bunch of beer cans and a half-empty bottle of vodka. "Let's check the other half," I suggested to Bob.

I drove the Engine slowly toward where the car front was pointing up, the head lights shining into the fog. The back part sat on the road, its sharp metal edges digging into the pavement. We looked in the door, shining our flashlights.

"There is someone lying there," Bob pointed out. We had found a man. His head lay on the pavement, and his feet were still propped up on the passenger front seat.

"I'll check this guy," I said, "you check for anybody else."

"Ok," Bob agreed. I knelt beside the man to see if he was breathing. His eyes opened.

"What happened?" he bellowed, the familiar alcohol breath stench pouring out of him.

"You have been involved in a car accident sir. Are you hurt?" I asked him.

"I don't think so," he responded. Bob called to me, "There is no one else in this half."

"Sir?" I asked, "was there anyone else riding with you?" "No... I don't think so," said the man. At that time the police arrived on the scene.

When the police officer reached us, he asked the man, "How are you feeling?"

"I feel great!" the patient responded. He repeated to the officer that he thought there had been no one else in the car.

"He *thinks*," I emphasized to the officer. He got the point.

"I will check the sides of the road," the officer said as he walked away. At that time Rescue Two arrived on the scene. I checked the patient from head to toe, and I couldn't find any injuries, except for a small cut on his hand. The medics came up beside me. One of them was a younger guy named Jake. He had dark hair and a moustache. There was a joke in the Department that we were all interchangeable: average build, 5'10", dark hair and a moustache.

"I can't find anything wrong with him, except a small laceration on his hand; and, he has ETOH on his breath." That was medical terminology for alcohol.

"Ok," Jake said.

"But, you should still put him on a back board," I suggested.

"We can take over here," Jake told me.

I walked back to the Engine and got out the tool kit. I went around to the front of the car, opened the hood and disconnected the battery. The headlights went out, and the sky went black.

In the dark, I saw a blue flash reflect off the front of the car. I turned around and saw another bright blue spark, about sixty feet away. It flared again, with a loud rumbling sound. "What is that?" I said out loud.

In the next flash, I saw a long pole lying across the road. Bob came running up to where I was standing, saying, "He must have knocked down the telephone pole. That must have been what cut his car in half."

Bob called on the hand radio, "Engine Three to dispatch. We have a pole down across the road, with live wires across Lone Pine Road, at Lake Shore. Contact the power company and have them come out."

"Message received, Engine Three." I pulled the Engine close to the wires, but not where we'd be in danger of contact. "Dispatch from Engine Three," Bob called out. "Engine Three," repeated dispatch.

"The wires are obstructing the road. We need a patrol car to block traffic on the other side of the wires," Bob ordered.

"Message received, Engine Three."

The police arrived soon after to help us blockade the accident scene. Curious people had started to gather, and we had to make sure that they did not endanger themselves. We also had to turn cars around that wanted to go through. It seems that someone always tries to get through, despite the road blocks.

"Engine Three, from dispatch." "Go ahead, dispatch."

"Engine Three, the power company has been notified and said there would be a three hour wait before they could get there."

"Ok, dispatch," Bob acknowledged with a hint of frustration. "Looks like we will be here for a while," I commented. A huge blue flash erupted just then. A wire shot across the road bouncing right towards us. Every bounce was accompanied by a bright blue spark. It fell far short of us, but it was spectacular to watch.

Over by the accident scene, I saw yellow flashing lights. That meant the tow trucks were picking up the severed car parts. I looked back at the electrical fireworks. There were two main areas where the discharges were most frequent and intense, on the side of the road and in the middle of the asphalt.

For four hours the wires gave us a light show before the power company arrived. They cut the power to the pole, and the large sparks finally stopped.

We had to check where the wires had been sparking, to see if any fire might have started. In the middle of the road we found a three foot circle that had burn marks. In the center of that was a puddle of melted asphalt, but there was no fire. I walked over to where the other wire rested on the side of the road. I couldn't believe what I saw. "Bob, look at this!" I called.

"What ya got?" he asked as he walked over.

We looked down on the shoulder, and in the sand was a deep hole, about six inches around and down out of sight. There was a cone of glass in the hole, made by the heat of the powerful electric discharges into the sand.

"That's something you don't see every day," I commented. It was still very hot. In fact, there was still some smoke coming rising out of the hole.

Bob said to me, "We'd better put some water in down there." I went to the Engine and pulled out the one inch hose off the reel. I sprayed water down the hole for about fifteen minutes, but none came back up.

"What do you think, Bob," I asked. "Is that enough water?" "Yeah, that's good."

I reeled the hose back up. When we checked the hole, it was no longer smoking. We shined the flashlight down into the cavity, but all we saw was black. We could not see the bottom. The glass had hardened as it cooled. The shape reminded me of water draining out of a sink. It appeared that our job was done here.

"Ok, Bob," I said. "Let's go home."

"Sounds good," he replied. On the radio he called, "Engine Three to dispatch, we are in service."

"In service received, Engine Three."

We left, with the power company in charge of the scene.

# Chapter 6 - Everyday Junk

It felt like I had just fallen asleep. I heard the familiar "Engine Three, you have a ----," but I couldn't hear what the dispatcher said.

Bob yelled, "We gotta go! Gun it!"

I pressed on the accelerator and the Engine lurched forward. To my horror, I noticed that the big apparatus room door was still closed. I slammed on the brakes, but too late. Blaaam! The metal door bowed, and the glass windows shattered with a crash. Pieces of glass rained onto the floor. Then part of the door collapsed on top of the Engine with a painful, loud bang. There was another crash and the sound of more broken glass.

The Engine came to a stop halfway out of the apparatus room as the crashing continued. After what seemed like forever, it got quiet. Bob and I looked at each other. I opened my mouth to ask what had happened, but part of the upper structure of the door broke free and smashed first on top of the Engine and then onto the floor. I could see and taste dust from the drywall that had just fallen too. I looked out the window and saw that most of the door was torn out. What wasn't broken free was bent out with the truck. I opened the Engine door and stepped down. I slid on broken glass. There was still a lot of dust in the air.

Bob turned to me and said, "Time to get up." "What?!" I answered, in confusion.

"Time to get up. You will be late for work." I saw Bob, but heard Wendy's voice. As my head cleared, I could see her beside my bed. I was at home.

"The alarm has been ringing for ten minutes!" she yelled.

"Ok, I'm up," I responded. As I woke, I realized it had just been another recurring dream. "What a relief," I muttered under my breath.

Wendy was pregnant with our second child, who was due in October. She had already been awake, puking in the bathroom thanks to morning sickness when the alarm had gone off.

"Are you all right?" I called to her.

"I will be," she answered. Then the phone rang.

"That will be Station One," I said to her. Whenever I got a call in the morning, it meant I was being sent to any station except for Station Three.

"I guess you will be going elsewhere," Wendy said to me as she ran back to the bathroom, her hand covering her mouth.

I answered the wall-mounted phone and, sure enough, it was from Station One.

"Let me guess," I preempted, "I'm going to Station One."

"Yes. Station One," came the response. "How did you know?" "I could tell by the sound of the ring," I joked. "I'll be there." While Wendy was in the bathroom, I cooked some corned beef hash with eggs. I dished out half to her and half to me. I was finishing my breakfast by the time Wendy came out of the bathroom.

"Your breakfast is ready," I said as she sat down.

"Thank you," she replied. One whiff of the corned beef almost immediately sent her running back to the bathroom, hand to her mouth. After finishing my breakfast, I went to the bathroom to ask, "Are you sure you're all right?"

"I will be," she said in a pained voice. "See you tomorrow."

"Anything I can do for you?" I asked.

"Just some privacy."

"Ok, see you tomorrow."

I wandered into my young son's bedroom to kiss him goodbye. I hoped I wouldn't wake him. At least give Wendy time to recover from morning sickness before Jimmy required all of her attention and energy.

I put peas in the monkey cage and pet the dog before getting in my truck and driving to Station One. On the way, I stopped for four deer crossing the road. It was almost a routine.

When I got to Station One it was 0730. My truck was the last vehicle to arrive. The parking lot was full, so I had to pull around back to park. I entered the station through the open apparatus room door. When I came into the living room and dining area, I was surprised that no one asked me to work for them so they could go early.

There were two reasons why we would get to work early. First, there was no excuse for being late. The Chief would say, "You had twenty-four hours to get to work. If you think you are going to have trouble getting here in the morning, then come in the night before and sleep here."

Once in a while some of us would do just that. It could be because a heavy snow storm was coming, or someone was arguing with their spouse.

The second reason I got to work early was so someone else could go home if I agreed to work for them. But today, no one asked. So, I went into the kitchen, got a cup of joe and sat at the kitchen table.

Across from me were two men and two women firefighters reading the newspaper. Beside me on my right was Bill, talking about his date the night before. On the left was Hal, talking about his two girls at home. Looking past Hal on my left was the living room, with the TV set tuned to the news broadcast. Men were sitting on the couch and chairs, watching TV or sleeping.

"Did you have a rough night?" I asked Hal.

"Yes," Hal said, rubbing his tired red eyes and stretching his long legs. "We were up all night."

"Well, Hal, if you want to go home early, go ahead," I offered.

"Ok, G.J. I will take you up on that." G.J. was another nickname that I had at the fire department. "You'll be in the back of the Rescue," Hal told me.

"Ok," I said.

Hal grabbed his shoes and disappeared out the door. I went into the bunk room and got my linens out of the locker and made my bed. I then went into the watch room to confirm what my assignment was for the day.

"You don't mind being third in the squad, do you?" the lieutenant asked me.

"No, that's what I expected." I usually was put as third on the Rescue if I was shipped in for the day. When we first started, the Rescues were originally called Life Squad Alpha and Beta. A few years later, they were changed to Squad One and Two. We added two more squads a few years after that, and the names were changed to Rescues One, Two, Four, Five and Nine.

The two rookies were busy in the apparatus room, going through all the trucks. At 0800, the shift going off-duty would pack up and leave. But one or two of them would hang around for a while, drink another cup of coffee or watch TV and b.s. with the guys.

I went out to the Rescue I was assigned to and ignored the "subby" (rookie), which is what we did to all of them until they were off probation. Thinking of the subby made me think back about my own time as the new guy. There was a tradition in the Department where the subby was sent to deal with an annual problem. Her name was Ada Barr. She was a crazy old woman that lived in a small bro- ken down house on Westphalia Street at the end of a long driveway up on the top of a hill. Everyone knew Ada Barr: Firefighters, Police,

Dispatchers and other township employees. Everyone except the brand-new employees, that is.

Ada Barr looked like the wicked witch of the west; short, skinny, drawn-in face, black growths on her nose and chin. She had no teeth that I could see, and had a distinctive voice. As soon as you heard it, you knew immediately who it was. Ada was a nice enough lady, I think, but at the least she was eccentric.

Every year at the end of October or the beginning of November, Ada would call 9-1-1 to ask where her turkey basket was. Every fall, a group of paid and volunteer firefighters, called the Goodfellows, collected money to help out the poor or those victims who had lost their house in a fire. We would stand in the intersections of West Bloomfield one day a year and give out a newspaper in exchange for a donation.

We'd use the money we collected to make turkey baskets consisting of a turkey, canned goods and other food items. It was a big basket. Somehow Ada knew about this and began calling 9-1-1, which went to dispatch, but also to the red fire phone at Station One.

When someone called 9-1-1 the fire phone would ring in the watch room. And by ring, I mean a loud buzzing that would knock you out of your bed. The day after my first Goodfellows' drive, the red fire phone rang. I was the closest, so I picked it up.

"9-1-1. What is your emergency?" the sweet voice of the dispatcher answered.

"Where is my turkey basket?" a horrible voice screeched.

"Hi Ada," came the dispatcher's immediate and polite reply.

"The baskets haven't been made yet, but…"

"When will I get my turkey basket!" Ada demanded. I wondered who the heck this woman was.

"It will be delivered as soon as they're done, Ada."

"I want my turkey basket now!"

"Ada the turkey basket will be there as soon as it's ready." The dispatcher must have been a saint to stay calm this long. She ended the phone call saying, "This is an emergency number, Ada. I have to hang up now."

Click. The phone went to dial tone. When I hung up the phone, everyone wanted to know if it was a run or not. I looked up and said, "it was someone named Ada Barr. Who is she?"

Everyone shook their head and said, "Oh, you'll find out soon enough," matter-of-factly and went back to what they were doing. On my next work day, I found myself parked in the fire utility truck atop a hill next to a tiny house. The paint was peeling badly on the ranch-style house, and one worn concrete step led to a screen door ridden with holes.

"What's the big fuss about dropping off this basket?" I wondered as I got out of my vehicle. I was about to knock on the door when I saw a pair of beady eyes glaring at me through the window on the main door.

"What do you want?" She hissed. I was taken aback, but calmly answered.

"I am from the Fire Department and I am here to deliver your turkey bas---."

The door flew opened and I found myself eye to eye with this woman. Incredibly, the hair on the back of my neck stood on end, and I felt something like terror as her claw-like hands snatched the basket from my grip. Before I could gather my wits about me, the door slammed shut and I was stood there alone...and trembling.

As I turned around, I stumbled down the cement step and found myself flat out on my back in the driveway. I thought of the knowing looks the guys at the station had given me. They knew what would happen, the bastards. I picked myself up, dusted off and got back in the truck. I survived my trial by fire.

The alert tones shook me out of my reverie. There was a long first tone, a shorter mid tone, and then a long, high station tone. As soon as the third tone started, we all knew it would be for Station One and headed to the watch room.

As I walked inside the door, the dispatcher said, "Station One, you have a person cut by an electric power saw at 3421 Western Run. Time out, 0914."

The lieutenant wrote the address on a piece of paper. We looked at the big wall map to find the cross streets. The section map was taken out to find the exact location of the address. Tom grabbed the section map and he, Rich and I headed to the rescue. Rich hopped in the driver's seat. Tom rode shotgun. I climbed in the back door and buckled myself into the jump seat.

Rich started the diesel engine and pulled the Rescue out as the apparatus room door finished opening. I was strapped in the jump seat, facing backwards. Not the most comfortable way to travel, especially when heading to an emergency at high speed.

There was always a high level of stress and anticipation of the injury and treatment sure to come. As we raced towards the scene, I sat in my seat, rocking back and forth. The shelves and cupboards were shaking, rattling and squeaking. Being in the back, you cannot anticipate the sharp sudden turns or the quick stops. You can't even hear the radio well.

The orange medical boxes slid side to side with each turn. With a sudden stop, we were there. I grabbed the orange medical box and the green oxygen bag. I also picked up the big radio duffle bag before opening the side door. Rich was there to help with the equipment. Rich walked with a limp, having crushed his ankles in a rock climbing accident years ago, but he was strong and had a great sense of humor. He was someone you could count on. I handed him the radio bag and hopped out.

We were parked in the driveway of a large two-story brick home. As we walked to the front door, a young woman appeared. She was visibly upset.

"My husband cut himself with an electric saw," she called to us.

"He is in the back."

We followed her to the back yard, around a deck that was being worked on. We had to step around a pile of old wood and a stack of new lumber. I could hear yelling as we got closer to the accident. The sound became louder as the injured man came into view. He was a young man in shorts with no shirt, lying on the grass. There was a circular saw resting in his lap. "I cut off my junk!" he screamed when he saw us.

Rich and I knelt next to him. In a steady voice, Rich said, "Calm down, sir. You will be all right."

I looked down and saw that his shorts were pulled up into the saw blade, against his "junk," as he called it. He did not have a cut on him, but the saw blade had pulled his shorts into the saw so tight
that it had caused an injury. On the ground between his legs were two small white pieces of flesh, with a string attached to each. The other end of the strings disappeared into his shorts. I realized then what I was seeing. The pressure had been so great, the poor guy's testicles had popped out like grapes.

"I cut off my penis!" he cried.

"No, it is all still there," I assured him. "Just relax and we will take care of you." Rich then told him, "Everything is intact. We will pack you up and take you to the hospital where they'll fix you up."

He started to yell again. "I have! I cut it off!"

"Just settle down. Your manhood is intact!" I interrupted, with a hint of exasperation.

Finally he relaxed enough for us to work on him. His testicles were lying on the grass, still attached to his groin by thin fleshy tubes. I freed the man's shorts from the saw blade. He was better able to relax, but was still in a lot of pain. Rich took a four-by-four gauze and carefully picked up the white pieces of flesh. I got another four-by-four and put it under the testicles.

Rich took the gauze from me, and I got a bottle of saline from the trauma kit. I opened it and poured saline on the gauze, wetting the testicles wrapped inside. The poor patient howled every time we moved him. By then, the ambulance arrived. The attendants brought the stretcher up next to us.

"Let's get him on the stretcher," I ordered.

The four of us picked the patient up, while Rich carefully held the man's privates. While we were wheeling the patient to the ambulance, Tom, with the clipboard, got the information needed for the report to relay to the hospital. We picked up the patient and put him in the back of the ambulance. Rich and I climbed in with him.

I pulled a bag of saline out of the cabinet with the IV tube. I also got an IV kit from the trauma box, which includes tubing, needles, bandages and alcohol skin sterilizers. I opened the package of saline with my teeth and then opened the tubing. I pushed the end of the tubing into the saline and opened the stopper, letting the liquid fill the IV tube.

Next, I got out the IV needle and the elastic tourniquet. I tightened the band around his arm, then felt for a vein. I found a likely candidate and pushed the needle in. When I got a blood flow, I pulled the needle out of the catheter. I attached the tubing to the catheter in his arm and started the IV.

Tom called the hospital and told them to have a surgery team ready. Also the ER doc ordered morphine as needed for pain. Shortly after the morphine was injected through the IV, our patient felt pain no more. Right then he was a happy man, despite the fact that his testicles were wrapped in gauze on the stretcher.

"So," Rich asked, "how did you injure yourself?"

"Well," he said, "I was working on my new deck. I was going to cut a piece of four-by-four wood. After I measured the wood, I took my saw, which is kind of old."

It was old, all right. I had seen it up close and noticed that it was all metal and well-used. The wires in the cord were even exposed.

The patient continued, "So, as I pulled the trigger, I felt a large electric shock, and my arm cramped. I couldn't control my arm. The saw was running full speed and my arm was contracting, pulling the saw closer and closer to my groin. I thought I was history, but my wife came out and unplugged the saw just as it cut into my shorts. My wife must have heard me scream. By the time the saw had stopped, it had grabbed my shorts and pulled them into the blade. Then it jammed and I heard a pop. Then pain," he paused. "It's a good thing my wife came out when she did. Can you imagine? Seeing yourself pulling an electric saw toward your own groin, the blade going full speed and there is not a thing you can do about it?"

"What a nightmare," Rich agreed with him. "At least it's over." We had just arrived at the hospital.

"Yes, it's over and I feel great!" he yelled as he was wheeled into the ER.

Rich said, "He's a happy camper now, but wait a few hours."

We gave the report to the nurses and the doctor. I helped Rich fill out the medical report at the nurses' station, which took about thirty minutes, while we flirted with the two nurses. Of course, that's why it took so long.

"Are you finished?" I asked Rich. "It is time to get into service." "I'm ready."

We walked through the emergency room and June, one of the nurses, grabbed Rich by the arm. "Why are you leaving so fast?" she asked. She was young and beautiful and very flirty.

We stopped walking and Rich answered, "We have to get back into service."

"Don't you have time for me?"

"Always time for you, June," Rich loved that kind of banter.

Didn't we all?

"Then why don't you accompany me to the med closet?" she suggested with a smile.

"Love to, darling, but we have to get back to the station."

"You can spare two and a half minutes can't you?"

We all laughed and then we walked out the door. "Bye, boys," June called out to us, waving.

"See you next run," we called back.

"I'll be here."

"I can't wait for the next run," Rich called back. Nurses often flirted with the firefighters, and vice versa. Some of the firefighters ended up marrying nurses, but Rich was already married with children. So was I. In fact, I was married to the most beautiful woman in the world (just in case she reads this).

# Chapter 7 - All in a Day's Work

"Something smells good," I said, walking into the kitchen at Station One. The subby was cooking ground beef. There are many good cooks in the fire department. I, however, was not one of them. Everyone took turns preparing meals, so sometimes they had to suffer through my cooking.

"Smells like tacos," Rich stated, rubbing his hands in anticipation.

"Nothing but the best for the men," replied the subby. "It will be ready in about ten minutes."

Rich and I started setting the table. By the time we were finished, the subby was putting the food out. "Lunch is ready!" he called.

Hal went into the office to get the Captain and the Chief. The Captain usually ate with us, but the Chief would normally go out for his meals. Chief Benson had come to us after a career in the Detroit Fire Department. He was the consummate professional, but he didn't have a sense of humor or a rapport with the guys. When they emerged from the office, the Chief headed out to his car, but Captain and Hal joined us.

The ground beef was on the table, along with salad, grated cheese, chopped up tomatoes and sour cream. The subby put the taco shells and tortillas alongside the rest of the food. I poured myself a soft drink and got my taco just right. I put the cheese in first, followed by the ground beef. That way, it melts the cheese. Then I added the shredded lettuce, followed by the tomatoes. As I reached for the sour cream, the sound of the fire tones went off.

"You've got to be #&%## kidding me!" someone screamed. He'd taken the words right out of my mouth.

It happened so often that a run would come in when we were eating. But this time, we didn't even get a bite. We waited for the tones to finish singing, which seemed to take a long time. If it was just a medical, the Rescue would go and everyone else would stay and finish lunch. If it was a PIA, the Engine would go with the Rescue. A fire meant we would all go.

"Dispatch to Station One. You have a possible house fire at 45532 Green Lawn. Neighbors have reported smoke showing."

"That's just across the street!" the Captain yelled.

We all ran to the watch desk. The lieutenant wrote down the address and looked it up on the wall map. Then someone handed him the section map. We ran to our respective vehicles, with Tom, Rich and I running to the Rescue.

Rich and I went in the back so we could suit up while Tom drove. The lieutenant and Hal were in the Engine. The subby and Bruce were on the Ladder. The Captain used to ride in the Engine and lead the way, but now he brought up the rear in his own Captain's car.

The diesel engines started simultaneously, as the big doors opened all at once. The automatic timer would close the doors after two minutes. The room filled with diesel exhaust as we pulled out. The fumes almost always made me sneeze.

We turned left, out onto the driveway apron, and the lieutenant called on the radio, "Engine One, Rescue One, Ladder One and Captain One responding to a possible house fire."

"Station One responding," said the dispatcher. "Be advised, other neighbors have called saying smoke visible. Also, the neighbor that called said there is an Indian family still in the house, and they don't speak much English."

"Message received, dispatch." We didn't have much time to put on our air packs and masks to get ready to go in to the house. Rich and I didn't say anything while we prepared. Then we came to a stop.

"Engine One to dispatch, all units are on scene of a three story house with a small amount of smoke visible from the lower front."

"Message received, Engine One."

Rich and I stepped out of the Rescue with the SCBA gear on our backs. I tightened the straps on my mask and reached back to turn on the regulator valve. A quick rush of air through the lines and into my mask, followed by a ringing sound, let me know that the SCBA was charged. We were now ready to go into the building.

The house was very large, basically a mansion. It was about four thousand square feet. As we reached the door, I could see the lieutenant in front of the large picture window.

He said, "Don't go in just yet."

I looked in the window, and there were about fifteen people sitting around a long dinner table. The smoke was not very thick. I lifted up my air mask and detected the smell of what seemed to be some sort of barbecue.

The lieutenant was staring in, too. He said, "What the hell?"

I took a closer look. The people were all dressed in brightly colored Indian clothes.

"There is no fire here," I said. The lieutenant grabbed his hand radio and called dispatch.

"Dispatch, there is no fire here. You can cancel all other responding units." He then said, "Rich, ring the doorbell."

Rich was taking off his mask as he pushed on the doorbell. I also took of my mask. We could hear ding, dong. No one at the table even looked up. Rich rang the doorbell again. No one looked up. I knocked on the window. A few people glanced our way, but then went right back to what they were doing.

"What's going on in there?" asked the lieutenant.

Looking in more carefully, I noticed there was a large grill, with a spit, and something was roasting on it. "They are having a barbecue in the house!" I yelled.

"They sure enough are," stated the lieutenant.

Rich tried opening the door, but it was locked. The lieutenant and I knocked on the window at the same time. Heads turned toward us again, and we waved them over. Incredibly, they ignored us and continued with what they were doing. Muttering some obscenities, the lieutenant knocked again and kept knocking until finally the door
opened. Smoke rushed out.

I could smell the barbecue, but it didn't smell good. In fact, it smelled like... well, I can't describe it exactly, but I can say that it was bad, in my opinion.

Standing in front of us was a small girl of about ten years old, long dark hair in a braid. She was dressed in colorful traditional Indian clothing, and sported a red dot on her fore- head.

"Can I help you?" she asked in heavily accented English. "I am the only one that can speak any English."

The lieutenant asked her, "Can we come in?"

"No sir," she answered.

"We are the Fire Department. We need to come in."

The little girl paused for a few moments and then asked us to wait. She walked over to the adults we had seen. "Oh, for heaven's sake!" exclaimed the lieutenant, disbelieving the apparent lack of concern the adults displayed.

The girl came back with a small, older man. "Father wants to know what you want?"

"Tell him to let us come in."

She talked to her father, and he waved us in. "Follow him," she said as she pointed into the house. We walked in behind him, the smoke immediately starting to burn my eyes.

The lieutenant asked the girl, "Why do you have a fire in the house?"

"We are fixing dinner," she answered. The father led us to the grill. It was quite large, and some animal was still roasting on the spit.

"What are you cooking?" I asked. She told us it was a goat. "You're not supposed to cook that in the house," the lieutenant sternly said. She said something to her father. He said something back to her.

She turned to us and asked, "Why not?"

"Because it is an outdoor grill, and it's made to cook outside!" the lieutenant yelled. "We will have to take it out of the house."

The lieutenant could see that the man still didn't understand. He tried to explain it again, saying "You can't have a grill fire in the house in America."

This seemed to come as much of a surprise to him as finding an active grill inside a house was to us. It was a case of mutual culture shock.

The lieutenant picked up the hand radio and called, "Lieutenant One to Engine One."

"Engine One," responded the driver.

"Bring in the fan and set it in the front door."

"I will bring in the fan, Lieutenant One."

I had to walk around the large table where the group sat to get into position to help. I pulled on the handle of the grill, goat and all, as the lieutenant pushed it towards the door. The door was opened when we got close enough, and we took it outside.

The crew of Engine One set up the fan in front of the main door. Someone pulled the starting rope, and the engine fired up the large blades of the fan. Air started to blow in through the front door. Someone went to open a window, after we realized they were all closed. It took about five minutes to clear the smoke out.

That is called positive pressure ventilation. We used to try to suck the smoke out by turning the fan around and drawing it out of the building. The fire departments did it that way for years, until it was discovered that pushing air in and forcing the smoke out through a small opening, like a window, was more efficient and a lot faster.

The air outside the window was smoky and filled our lungs and nostrils with retched goat perfume.

"What a great fragrance," I said between coughs, as we pulled the grill with the goat around to the side yard.

The lieutenant went back into the house to get report information and to try to explain again the need to grill outside. Engine One crew and Rescue One crew shut off the fan and packed it back in the truck. We waited in front of the door until the lieutenant came back out.

As he stepped out of the front door, he said, "Now that's something you don't see every day."

"Or smell," someone else piped up. That was one of the exciting things about West Bloomfield, with all of the different cultures. You just never knew what to expect.

"Ok, let's get back and eat our lunch," said the lieutenant, as he picked up the hand radio.

"Dispatch from Lieutenant One; all units are in service."

"In service received, Lieutenant One," answered the dispatcher. We walked to our trucks, taking off our equipment as we went. I climbed into the back of Rescue One. The truck started to pull ahead, and I took off my fire coat. I hadn't realized how hot and sweaty I had become. My blue shirt was soaked.

Unexpectedly, the alarm tones went off, causing me to jump in my seat. "It'd better be for Three's or Four's!" someone in the front cried. Rich and I started throwing our fire coats back on as the tones stopped and we knew it was for us.

"Station One, you have another possible house fire at 3224 Round Lane. Round Lane is in your vicinity."

"Ok, dispatch, I know where it is," called the lieutenant over the radio. We had already been on Round Lane when the run was dis- patched. As the name suggested, the road was one big loop. I threw all my gear back on as we traveled around the circle, not finishing before we came to a stop.

"Engine One, Rescue One, Ladder One on scene and smoke showing."

I heard the hissing sound of the air brake as Rich and I finished getting on our gear. We hopped out as we were clipping our fire coats closed. I looked up and saw a large, white single-story house with a brick front and a large circular cement driveway. There was smoke billowing out of the eaves.

The large picture window in front was black with smoke. You could see the pressure of the hot, sooty gas trying to escape. It seemed that the whole house was pulsing; expanding and contracting like a giant heart. With each beat, a jet of black smoke was forced out over each window, under the eaves.

"Lieutenant One reporting a working house fire. Have Engine Three respond."

"Message received, Lieutenant One. Engine Three, respond to 3224 Round Lane," called the dispatcher.

I never heard Engine Three respond, because Rich and I were preparing to go in the house. Engine One had already pulled out the two and one half inch hose bundles and had stretched the three inch line to the hydrant. Dropping hose line from the fire scene and stretching line to the hydrant is called a reverse lay. That is how we did it in those days.

The problem with the reverse lay is that the engine was at the hydrant and might be a long way off from the fire. So, we would have to pull off the equipment we thought we might need and lay the two one and a half inch bundles in front of the house. Then we stretched two and a half inch line to the hydrant.

Half way through my career, we changed tactics and began using forward lay. Forward lay is first, find the hydrant, (which was indicated on our maps), then stop in front of the hydrant and drop the three or four inch line with a firefighter, and finally, drive the truck to the fire scene. Meanwhile, the firefighter that was dropped at the hydrant connects the hose to the hydrant. Then the Engine stretches the hose from the hydrant to the front of the structure. At this fire, however, we did the reverse lay.

As we watched the line from the hydrant and Engine fill up with water, the lieutenant ordered, "Get ready to go in!" We could see a family standing on the sidewalk. The lieutenant yelled to them.

"Is everyone out of the house?"

"I think so," the man responded. "I believe my other son is at his friend's house but I'm not sure."

"Great," muttered the lieutenant. "There might be someone in the house. Also, the fire is in the bedroom."

By that time, the water had straightened the two and a half inch line and the one and a half inch line was connected via a Y connector. Rich and I were holding the inch and one half line; me in front and Rich behind. The line stiffened in my hands and water dripped out the nozzle. I checked the nozzle to make sure it was not plugged by twisting it open. Water rushed out, and I closed it, satisfied that all was in order.

"I'll open the door, and you go in!" yelled the lieutenant. We both nodded. The lieutenant tried to open the door, but it was locked. The lieutenant said, "Johnson, kick it open!"

I expected a lot of resistance, so when I kicked the door I lifted my leg and put all my weight into it. To my surprise, my foot met with little resistance, shattering the jamb and sending splinters of wood exploding into the air. As the door slammed open, I fell forward through the entry, landing on my knees and taking Rich with me. Smoke poured out of the house. Both of us had been caught off guard.

"Well," said Rich, "I guess we are ready to go in."

His voice was muffled through the rubber mask, making it difficult to understand, but I knew what he meant. He tapped my back, and we started in.

We began crawling into the house, dragging the hose line with us. The farther we went, the darker it became. Soon, all the light was gone and it was pitch black. With each breath, I could hear the air swish in my mask, and could also detect a slight odor of wood smoke.

I heard Rich's muffled yelling to me, but I could not understand what he was saying. I stopped and turned to listen to him. He tapped my left shoulder and said, "I just ran into the couch, so the bedroom is that way."

"Ok!" I yelled back. We continued crawling and took a left at the couch. We felt our way into a hall. It was getting hot. We got down a little lower. I felt a doorway on my left. I pushed my head through and could see a faint yellow-red glow. "I see it!" I yelled.

Rich responded, "Throw some water on it."

I opened the nozzle and a burst of water shot out, pushing me back a little. The water splashed back off what I was spraying, covering my mask. The glow was gone. That was too easy, I thought. We crawled a few feet further and felt a large opening.

"It's a fireplace!" I yelled. "This is not the fire. Let's keep going!" Rich patted me twice on the back to let me know he understood. I felt along the fireplace and we went into another hallway. The radio in my coat pocket was screaming. Someone shouting orders, firefighters and dispatchers answering.

Sirens wailing. But in the fire, we were alone. We made our way further down the hall.

Rich tapped my back and said, "It's getting hotter."

I nodded in agreement; it was significantly hotter. We came to the end of the hall. In front of us was a doorway. Inside, I could hear crackling and saw a large red glow in front of us. I started to turn around to tell Rich, but he patted me on the back to tell me he saw it. We moved ahead into the large bedroom.

The fire was a blur, but it came into focus as we got closer. There were flames from the ceiling down to the floor. They had even spread to the bed. Almost all of the room was filled with flames. I opened the nozzle and a jet of water shot out. I pointed it to the bed for a moment, then to the ceiling and then to the floor.

I couldn't tell where the fire was coming from. So I sprayed water all around the room. Just then I heard a crash! Someone had broken out a window next to us. Glass fragments clanked off our helmets. Another window shattered as I kept putting water on the fire. Finally the glow started to subside, then went out.

The smoke was clearing quickly. A fan had been put in front of the door, and when the windows were broken in, the air from the fan forced the smoke out. I could see now, and it was cool enough to stand up. My air tank alarm rang as I got to my feet, meaning my air supply was almost out.

The bed had a charred blanket with what looked like a body under it. I went up to the bed to check, lifting up the blanket and revealing a dead pile of clothes. I laughed to myself as I let it back down. "This room must belong to a teenager," I said.

By that time, Bob had arrived. He and another firefighter were doing a search to make sure no one was in the house. I started to walk out, because when the bells on my air tank went off, it meant I only had five minutes before my air ran out. I took two steps toward the door when I heard a scream behind me.

I whipped around and saw Bob jumping away.

"What is it?" I yelled to Bob.

"It's a body! I stepped in a body!"

I walked to where Bob was standing, wondering what he meant. Then I saw. Beside the bed was a badly burned body with most of the clothes burned off and a boot-sized bloody hole in the abdomen. The body was unrecognizable.

"I guess you found Aunt Sally," said the lieutenant, who had just walked in. My air ran out, so I pulled off my mask. Then Rich's tank alarm rang, and he took off his mask as well. The air was clear, so it was ok to breath for a while.

"Aunt Sally!" Bob cried, still horrified.

"After you went in, the family remembered that no one had accounted for Aunt Sally. That must be Aunt Sally," he said gesturing to the charred body. "They were afraid she might have started the fire. She was a smoker," the lieutenant added as he looked down at the body.

It was charred on the outside, but the inside was clearly human. I could see the intestines, stomach and other organs. She was dead before she was burned. You could tell this because there was no bleeding.

"Good job, Bob, you found Aunt Sally," I joked, trying to lighten the mood for a moment. Bob looked up and back down, not saying anything.

The lieutenant turned to me and said, "You and Rich go and get some rest and water."

"Yes sir," Rich replied. I then realized I was dog tired. As we passed him, the lieutenant said, "Good work in the fire."

"Thanks, Lieu," I said as we walked out. It's not often you get a compliment, so you'd better take it when you can. Rich and I walked to the rest station near where Engine Three was parked. There were two medics and some volunteers with water, coffee and donuts. Rich and I sat down on the ground and got a bottle of water.

A medic came up to us and asked, "Are you guys all right?"

"Yeah, fine."

"Well, I need to take your vitals."

"Ok," Rich said, sticking his arm out. I did the same.

"That was a good stop," the medic said as he put on the blood pressure cuff. He pumped up the cuff as I felt the familiar squeezing on my arm.

"It's good," he said. "120/80."

"Perfect," I muttered, not really feeling it.

He took Rich's BP and then sat down with us. After about twenty minutes, Rich and I had recovered and went back into the house. The whole inside was covered with a layer of black soot.

It was always strange to me when I reentered a building after I put out a fire. Everything looked so different. In the fire, I couldn't see anything. I could only feel my way around. The picture in my mind looked quite different than what I would see after. I went up to the fireplace where I had put out the contained fire. It was a lot smaller area than it had seemed at the time. Also, the long hallways were not so long after all. But they were now black with soot.

I went back into the bedroom. The body was still there. It didn't look real, but it smelled real enough. Nothing like the smell of charred human flesh. After the ME left with the body, we had to overhaul the site.

There's not much worse than having to come back and put out a fire again because of a rekindle. We were there for three more hours, using pike poles to pull down ceiling tiles and wallboard, smoldering pieces of cloth and furniture. Men with hoses wet down hot spots. Then the lieutenant let the owners into the house to see the damage. That's when I walked out.

We broke down and rolled up the hoses. When the lieutenant was finished with the family, we finally went back to the station. You might think we were done at that point, but no! We still had to wash the hose and put it in the hose dryer while someone else washed the trucks. Others serviced and put away the equipment, repacked the trucks, and washed the floor. Only then were we finished.

Engine Three went back to Station Three, and we were ready for lunch. Only thing was, it was dinner time now and the lunch food we'd abandoned was old and cold. So, the watchman cook went out and got pizza. While we were cleaning off the dinner table, the Captain came out of his office. He had been at the fire somewhere, but
I hadn't seen him.

He said, "I just got a call from the home owner. He claims that because we took too long to get to the fire, about ten minutes, his aunt died."

"Really?" came our incredulous response. "But Cap, we were already in the neighborhood!"

"It took less than a minute to get there!" said the lieutenant, his face turning red as his blood pressure shot up in frustration.

"I know, John. The dispatchers are retrieving the tapes, so don't worry about it. That's *my* worry."

"Unbelievable!" I said to Rich.

The Engineer of Engine One spoke up. "That was a damn good stop!"

Everyone at the table spoke up at the same time, complaining and saying "good stop."

Sometimes ours was a thankless job.

# Chapter 8 - Tragedy and Comedy

Later that afternoon, I sat down to watch the TV news, as I planned out something for the station party we would have between Thanksgiving and Christmas. The kids and families of the crews would gather at the station for some holiday fun. I would perform a marionette show and "Santa" would ride in on one of the Engines, ready to spread holiday cheer. My boys looked forward to it, so I was preparing for this year's celebration while I had the chance.

No sooner had I settled into a soft recliner, my notepad in hand, when the tones went off. As they sounded, men were hopefully chanting, "Threes! Threes! Threes!"

"Station One, you have a possible suicide in the woods on Pontiac Trail. South side of the road, just east of the railroad tracks. Time out, 1917."

"Rescue and the Engine go, Ladder stays here," ordered the lieutenant. I climbed into the back of the Rescue. Tom drove and Rich rode shotgun.

The doors opened as the diesel engines roared to life. We started to roll. I could smell the fumes, which made me sneeze. It had become part of my routine. "Gesundheit," came the automatic response from the front.

"Thank you," I responded. We passed through the apparatus room door as the sirens wailed. The Engine followed us.

"Engine One, Rescue One responding."

"Responding received, at 1919."

We pulled out north on Orchard Lake Road. It was still light out-side, but the sun was starting to go down. I crawled up between the two front seats as we reached the intersection at Pontiac Trail. I was supposed to be belted into the jump seat in back, but I always wanted to see what the situations were so I could decide what equipment to bring out. Besides, I didn't like riding backwards.

As we slowed down, the traffic light turned green. That didn't happen too often. It seems like the light always shone red for us. We turned west on Pontiac Trail and accelerated as the vehicles pulled to the side of the road. It was a short ride until the railroad tracks came into view.

We slowed down when we saw a man standing on the left side of the road, his face covered in blood. We quickly came to a stop. I pulled the trauma kit out and hopped down from the back.

When I saw the injured patient more clearly, I was shocked. Rich and Tom were surrounding the man, whose face was missing. It had been completely torn off, leaving a mess that dripped blood onto the ground.

The man was in shock and started to fall. We all reached for him and helped him to sit down. As we examined him, we found that he had no eyes, no nose and no lower jaw. Ragged pieces of flesh were hanging off his skull. The only thing that was left was a tongue sticking out of a bloody hole that was once his face.

He tried to talk, but with no lips or jaw, it made understanding him impossible. His tongue was hanging out of the bloody cavity, waving up and down and making guttural noises. "Glop, glop, glop," was all we could hear.

It was clear that his airway was open, and the bleeding had mostly stopped. Tom tried to reassure him. "We've got you. You're in good hands."

I reached into the trauma box and pulled out a large dressing and a roll of gauze. I placed the dressing on the wound and wrapped the gauze around his head to keep the dressing securely in place. When
I finished, his head was completely wrapped with gauze, except the hole where his mouth used to be. The police had just arrived.

"His name is Shaun Baxter," the police officer told us. "His mother called and said he had a shot gun and was suicidal," the officer reported. I noticed there were other police officers walking in the woods nearby. I wasn't sure what they were looking for.

I took out a bag of saline and an IV kit. I opened the kit and ripped the plastic cover off the bag of saline. I spiked the end of the IV tubing into the bag of saline and set the needles next to him. I opened an IV needle and took an alcohol swab and cleaned the IV site on his arm.

"We are going to start an IV, so you will feel a little poke," I told Shaun. He tried to answer, but it just sounded like "glop, glop, glop!"

His tongue flapped up and down. I pushed the needle under his skin and got a blood return. Then I bled the air out of the tubing and stuck it in the pulled-out needle opening. I opened the drip to sixty drops per minute. "Let's give him some morphine."

Rich handed me the preloaded syringe and I injected the proper amount into the IV. Almost immediately, he relaxed. The ambulance had arrived and the crew brought the stretcher next to us. We lifted him onto the stretcher and rolled it to the back of the ambulance.

Tom came up to me and asked, "Do you mind driving the Rescue to the hospital? I would like to go with him in the ambulance."

"Sure, I'll drive the truck."

Tom hopped in the back of the ambulance with Rich, and I shut the door. They sped off with their lights flashing. I stood there watching for a moment, then turned to head back to the Rescue.

I was a guest at Station One, you might say. So they usually let the visitors from other stations drive the truck to the hospital. I was walking to the Rescue when a voice came out of the woods.

"I found a shotgun!" The police officers started running down to the where the voice had come from. I had a few minutes before I had to leave for the hospital, so I headed over to the woods where the police had gathered. They were standing under a tall maple tree, looking and pointing up. I followed their gaze and saw blood and pieces of flesh splattered on a low hanging branch.

"Here is a note," one officer called.

The others circled around him and read the letter. I can't say what the note said, but it was clearly a suicide attempt. The police said he tried to kill himself by putting a 12 gauge shotgun under his chin. When he pulled the trigger, he must have flinched, causing him to almost miss.

"Ok. Now I know," I thought to myself as I walked back up to the truck. I got in and drove to the hospital, pondering what had just happened. When I reached the hospital, Tom and Rich had already finished the paperwork and were standing outside the emergency entrance.

"What took so long?" Tom asked me.

"I found out what happened. He tried to kill himself with a shotgun and missed."

"That will change his life," said Rich. Then he said "Do you know what we are having for dinner?"

When I shook my head in response, Rich answered his own question. "Open-faced sandwiches."

We paused for a moment, then broke out laughing. Rich was always saying things like that. But making jokes about bad situations helped to ease a stressful day. We arrived at Station One at 0030. Everyone who had not been on the run was in their bunks except John, who was still watching TV.

"I should go to bed," I said, "but I might just watch some TV too."

I sat down on the recliner, and Rich and Tom sat on the couch. When we had runs like that, we would stay up for a while to unwind. Trying to fall asleep now, even though we were tired, would have been difficult at best.

The alarm for the watchman woke me up. I was still sitting on the recliner. We had been so busy I hadn't even made my bunk. Men were starting to gather around the table.

"The coffee is ready," said the watchman. I got up and stood in line to get my coffee. It was still quiet. Everyone was half asleep. Rich always told good stories, and he started telling the men about our run.

"Yeah, he took a shotgun and blew his face into the tree. Do you know what we are having for meals tomorrow? Open-faced sandwiches." Everyone laughed or groaned. There was a hockey game replay on TV. That gave me an idea, so I piped up, "Look! They're having a face off."

Everyone laughed again. Then others started to try to make open-face jokes. That is how we coped with the grim situations we had to deal with. If you thought about some of these incidents and the victims too much, you wouldn't survive long in this job.

It was my family that kept me sane through the years. I cherished the time I was able to spend with them. Sometimes Wendy would come by the station with the boys in tow when I was working. They loved to climb on the equipment and hang with the crew when they could. Fortunately, the Department never discouraged this practice. It helped keep morale up to know we could sneak some extra time in with our families.

What may not be surprising is that my oldest son, Jimmy, wanted to follow in my footsteps. After high school he completed Fire Fighter school and Paramedic training at Schoolcraft Community College. He was able to get a paid-on-call job locally, but there just weren't any permanent openings in the departments around here.

He ended up joining the Air Force and serving our country. Although I'm proud of him and what he's doing, I still think he would have made an excellent fire fighter. I thank God every day for the family I was privileged to head.

# Chapter 9 - Dark Times

Something you learn as a first responder is that you're never home free until you're in your car and more than halfway home. With only thirty minutes until 8:00, when I could leave, the tones went off. Of course, it was for Station One, which is where I was that day.

"You have got to be kidding me!" someone yelled, more than a little frustrated.

Dispatch called out, "You have a child hit by a car at 5557 Maple Avenue. Time out, 0735."

I set my coffee on the table and walked to the Rescue. I didn't even hear the radio or smell the fumes or sneeze. I just climbed in the back and sat down backwards. I turned over my shoulder and said to the two in front, "I hope it's nothing."

"Rescue One, be advised police reporting that you'd better step it up. A very serious injury involving a child," the dispatcher said in a distressed voice.

My heart sank and all lightheartedness left me. Nothing bothered me more than injured or sick children. I sat back in my chair and waited for the Rescue to get to the scene.

"Rescue One on scene," I heard, as I quickly scrambled out of the back with the trauma box. I looked up the circular driveway to where a black car sat in front of a white garage. I heard screaming coming from behind the car. A police officer stuck his head up over the vehicle and yelled, "Over here!"

He waved for us to come. We all ran to the back of the car. There was a girl of about two years old, lying on the driveway behind the right rear wheel. A man, woman and police officer were kneeling over her. I set the box down and knelt beside her as the police officer gave up his spot for me. The girl was unconscious, blood running out of her nose and ears. I opened her eyes and saw they were unequal and semi-dilated.

"Let's get her in the Rescue!" Tom called out. Rich scooped up the girl, and we all raced to the truck. I opened the back and we hopped in. Her mother and father followed, but stopped at the door. Her mother was sobbing bitterly.

Rich yelled, "Greg, you drive! We've got to go right now!"

"Ok," I said as I ran to the police officer that had just arrived, "I need your help! I need you to lead me out of here."

"What hospital?" the officer asked.

"St. Andrews." "Ok. Let's go."

I needed his help because it was a long winding subdivision. I had ridden in back of the Rescue on the way in, so I had no idea how to get back to the main road, and there was no time to figure it out. The officer hopped in his squad car, and I went over to the Rescue to close the side door. Tom, the toddler cradled in his arms, looked up and sadly said, "She's history."

I closed the side door and went to the driver's side, where I was met by the father. He said, "I'm going too."

"Ok," I said, "get in the passenger side."

He ran over to the passenger door and got in. The police car pulled in front of us, blue lights flashing, and I followed behind, turning on my red lights. I followed the officer through the confusing subdivision until he led me to Northwestern Highway. The police car turned to go back to the tragic scene as we continued on toward
the hospital. The morning rush was just getting started, and the road was crowded and slow. The traffic came to a complete stop.

"We'll never get through!" cried the distraught father.

"Oh, we'll get through," I assured him, pulling onto the left shoulder and speeding along the gravel next to the highway. We accelerated past the traffic, siren blaring, stones, gravel and dust flying in our wake. We came to the road construction site that was causing the delay.

The road became fairly clear after that. The rest of the traffic moved to the sides of the highway. As we were getting closer to the hospital, the father began to speak.

"My wife was backing out of our driveway. I saw my little girl running to her mother in the car. I ran after her, but it was too late. She fell under the tire and the car ran over her head. I could hear the crunch," he told me as tears streamed down his face. I took a deep breath, trying to hold back my own tears.

It didn't take long to get to the hospital from there, but two minutes seemed like hours. As we pulled into the emergency entrance, we were met by four nurses, two doctors and two orderlies. I left the engine running after I pulled into the emergency stall. I ran to the back of the truck and opened the rear door. The father followed.

The nurses and doctors met us as Tom climbed out of the Rescue. He handed over the child to a nurse. They rushed the lifeless little girl to a trauma room where they worked on her. The father was taken to another room with a nurse. The only thing we could report to the staff was what the father said had happened. We didn't even have time to learn her name.

Nothing had changed with the girl since leaving her home. She was still comatose; her eyes were unequal and dilated. Blood and spinal fluid was dripping from her nose and ears, but she was still breathing.

Rich, Tom and I sat at the nurses' desk for quite a while without saying anything. Finally, Rich started the paperwork. The nurses had the information for our report, which took about twenty minutes to finish. As we got up to go home, a doctor walked out of the trauma room. We could tell by his face that it wasn't good news. "I had to call it," he told us. "Time of death 0902."

"Thanks, Doc," I answered sadly. He walked away towards the room with the girl's father.

We strode out the emergency room door back to the Rescue. We got in our truck and headed back to the township. It was a quiet ride back. No jokes or kidding around like we usually did after a particularly difficult run. I took this one hard, partly because I was about to have another kid of my own. I couldn't imagine what it would feel like to lose a child. How would the parents deal with the loss? In my experience with tragedies like this, the marriage usually breaks up.

I had to get my mind right. I just wanted to get home and hug my wife, our son and the one still inside her. We reached the border of our township. Rich picked up the mic, keyed it and said, "Rescue One in service."

"In service received, Rescue One." A short pause followed; then, "Rescue One, you have a PIA."

"No!" we all screamed.

"Truck verses a motorcycle at the intersection of Maple and Orchard Lake Roads. Time out, 0921."

Without a word, Rich flipped on the lights and siren. For a while, at least, we had to forget the run we just had. It was a short ride from where we were to the accident site, only about two miles. I sat back in my chair and tried to calm myself for the upcoming run.

"Engine One on scene," I heard over the radio. Engine One had the next day's crew. We were technically off the clock. Don't get me wrong, we'd get overtime pay, but we would rather be at home.

"Engine One reporting serious injuries." "Rescue One has the message." Rich called over the radio, "Rescue One on scene."

It was always tough to anticipate what we would have when you rode in back. There was one small window on the passenger's side, but of course, we pulled up to the scene with the accident on the driver's side. I couldn't see anything, so I asked the guys, "What do we need?"

"Just the trauma box for now," Rich answered. We came to a stop right next to an eighteen wheeler semi. The crew of Engine One was at the back of the dirty silver trailer.

There were also two patrol cars, their blue lights flashing. One was on the intersection, directing traffic. The other was parked beside Engine One in the middle of Maple Road, blocking the roadway.

We rushed to the back of the very large tractor trailer. There was a young man lying between the two rear tires.

The lieutenant met us and reported, "We have a badly injured man. Witnesses said that the light turned red when the truck stopped. The victim was on a motorcycle five cars behind. He got impatient, drove around the traffic and crashed into the back of the truck."

As we were being filled in, we began working on the patient. "We need a backboard and a C collar!" I yelled. Someone from Engine One got up and ran to the Rescue to get them. I was at the man's head. The patient was unconscious and was laboring to breathe. I noticed he didn't have a helmet on.

"Was he wearing a helmet?" I asked.

"No, they said he was not wearing a helmet when he crashed," the lieutenant responded. The Rescue crew for today's shift had just arrived in a FD pickup truck.

"I need the airway kit," I called to them. I was going to intubate the patient while the others examined him.

"Let's get him out first," someone suggested.

"Good idea," I agreed. "I've got the head. Let's pull him towards me." The long back board was already in position. There were five of us; me at the head, one on each shoulder and one on each leg.

"On three," I called out. "One, two, three!" We lifted him up together, with me holding his head and neck still.

"Down on Three." I counted again. "One! Two! Three!"

We set him softly on the board. Someone handed me the laryngoscope, and I proceeded to put the tube in his trachea. I saw it go between the vocal chords.

I used a ten cc syringe to fill the bulb with air to hold it in place. Someone handed me a bag mask. I hooked it to the tube and squeezed it, putting air in his lungs. I put a stethoscope to his chest, listening as I squeezed the mask again. I heard strong breath sounds.

"Sounds good!" I announced. I listened to his lungs again, and I heard some gurgling in each lung. "He must have broken ribs. He has bilateral pneumothorax." I knew that without immediate treatment, his lungs would likely collapse. One of the Unit Two Rescue crew members was starting an IV.

"We will take it from here, if you want."
"Sounds good to me," I agreed. We changed places with the new crew. I looked at the patient as he was lifted onto the stretcher. He had two broken femurs, open fractures of both lower legs, and an open fracture of his right forearm. When his bones broke, the sharp end cut through the tissue. Nasty injuries. Tom and Rich had bandaged and splinted the fractures.

The ambulance had arrived, so we picked the patient up and put him on the stretcher and then into the back of the vehicle. We made sure that the Unit Two crew was up to speed on the patient's status. Then Mark from Unit Two said, "We've got this. You guys go on home."

I said, "Thanks, guys!" I was about to hop out when I noticed blood being exhaled through his breathing tube. Mark suctioned out the tube.

"Before you go," Mark asked, "will you listen to his lungs?" "Sure." I grabbed the stethoscope from around my neck and placed it on his chest. "Left lung, no breath sounds," I told him. Right lung diminished breath sounds."

One lung has collapsed and the other is about to," Mark summarized with concern. The Unit Two crew had already hooked him up to the heart monitor. His heart rate was tacky.

"PVC's," (premature ventricular contractions) I said as I hopped out. I closed the back door as the ambulance sped off, kicking up stones as it left. I watched as it turned out of sight. I went back to the accident scene where Tom, Rich and the rest of Unit One were working.

"That guy is messed up," Rich said.

"Yes he is. I don't think he will make it." The police were measuring the scene in case he died.

"He was only nineteen," someone said. "Not a good start to the day," I stated.

Lieutenant then said to us, "He never even slowed down. I wonder why he didn't see this big rig? The police said he was going about 40 miles per hour when he impacted the truck. His body hit the underride guard mounted on the back. The bike slid under the truck, dragging him under too."

"That explains the injuries." I said. "I don't think he's going to make it."

"Well," the lieutenant said, "you guys are off duty now. Take the pickup back to the station and go home. And don't forget to fill out the overtime sheet."

"Ok, Lieu." Rich, Tom and I walked to the pickup and got ready to leave. The Unit Two boys had parked the truck between two police cars, leaving the lights flashing. We were maneuvering to get out from the between the patrol cars when a black car sped past us. It slammed on the brakes and came to a stop right in front of the accident scene.

Both the doors, driver's and passenger's, flew open. A man and woman jumped out and ran over to the accident site. "That must be the parents," Rich said as we pulled away.

As we arrived at Station One I thought to myself, "not a good day." We pulled into the empty station, which had an eerie feel to it. We didn't have to do paperwork because the Unit Two boys took over the run and they would have to do it. We stepped out of the truck as the doors came down. We didn't say much as we went to our cars, each man lost in his own thoughts.

I can't really imagine what it must have been like for the parents to deal with the death of their children. The closest we ever came to knowing was when my oldest son was only one or two years old. He was pretty sick, having trouble breathing and dealing with lots of phlegm.

The doctor wanted to test him for cystic fibrosis. For one agonizing week we waited for the results of that test, knowing that the results had the potential to change our lives forever. It came back negative, leaving us feeling relieved and grateful to God once again.

Maybe it's the nature of the job we did, but most of the crew had a religious faith. There were one or two exceptions, including one guy who was the most devout atheist I'd ever known. There's something about watching people die, or the miracle of someone living when it defies all logic that strengthens your belief in something greater than yourself. Without my faith, it would have been difficult to work this job for thirty years.

# Chapter 10 - Laughing Keeps You Sane

I enjoyed working at Station Four the most. It was just a great group of people and a more or less manageable pace. One slow day, we were sitting around the kitchen table, drinking coffee. There were three other firefighters talking to me about the last shift's runs when

Rich spoke up. "Tell the guys about how you fished with the RC (radio controlled) motor boat."

"Ok," I started, "I have a very large bass in my pond. I call him Cecil Fishy. He is tame; I feed him worms out of my hand."

"Can I come over and fish?" Paul interrupted.

"Better yet," I said, taking a sip of coffee, "just stick your hand in the water holding a worm. If you can keep your hand in the water when he strikes, I'll give you fifty dollars." I continued explaining, "Cecil doesn't nibble; he strikes your hand! He hits the worm some of the time."

To make a point, I lifted up my hand to show the scrapes on my finger and thumb. "He doesn't have any teeth, but he hits hard and his fish lips have ridges that will do this," I indicated my scars. "You can't see him coming, then he strikes and scares the shit out of you."

After another sip of coffee I continued. "Anyway, Cecil was named after the baseball player Cecil Fielder. I was feeding him worms when I got an idea; I could go trolling with my radio control boat. I rigged the boat with a small fiberglass pole, a line and a hook. I didn't want Cecil to get caught, so I asked Wendy to throw worms into the pond at the dock, while I put the boat in the water with a baited hook."

"Did you catch anything?" someone asked.

"Just wait," I said, stringing them along. They were all looking at me intently as I continued. "I put the boat in the water while Wendy kept Cecil busy at the other end of the pond. As soon as the boat was in the water and was trolling, Wendy yelled, 'Cecil is gone!'

Immediately there was a tug on the boat, then another. Suddenly, the whole boat disappeared under the water in the blink of an eye. A few seconds later, the bow of the boat came to the surface. It bobbed once or twice, then bloop! It was gone again.

I got in my paddle boat and headed out to where the little RC boat sank. I could see the boat on the bottom of the pond, near a drop off. All of a sudden, the boat was pulled and it dropped off the edge and disappeared out of sight. After a few minutes, it was clear it was a lost cause. I paddled back to the dock where I found Cecil waiting for more worms."

The men were laughing as the tones went off. We heard, "Station Four, you have a possible suicide at 5631 Scott Road in Zox Sub. Time out, 0801."

We rushed to the watch room to look on the wall map. It was now shift change, which made things confusing. When calls came in at these times, we could end up with two crews crowding around the map. Also we may not have received our assignments or have had the chance to check out our trucks and make sure they were ready for runs.

I found out that I was driving the Rescue. Rich was riding shotgun and Paul was in back. I thought to myself, not another suicide! I hadn't even finished my coffee.

Lights and sirens blaring, we pulled out the door onto Greer Road and east to Zox sub. It only took two minutes for us to arrive at the small house. A woman was waiting for us at the side of the road.

"He's upstairs," she told us. "I heard a loud gunshot. I haven't been up there," she added. She didn't sound all that surprised.

The three of us entered the house and climbed the stairs. Rich was carrying the clip board, Paul had the trauma kit and I had the LIFEPAK heart monitor. The first room that we came to at the top of the stairs was the correct room.

I was first in. Immediately, the terrible smell of gun powder mixed with brain matter and blood greeted me. Brain matter has a special smell of its own.

I looked up from the floor, knowing what I'd find. A young man of about seventeen was lying across a bed, a shotgun on the floor nearby. Rich and Paul had followed me into the room. We just stood there for a moment, knowing there was nothing we could do to help him. I looked up and saw red flesh splattered across the ceiling, surrounding a large hole in the plasterboard, where the shotgun blast had impacted it. There were also skull fragments stuck in the ceiling.

"Well, I guess we should hook him up to the monitor," I suggested, as we looked over the victim. Paul attached the monitor leads. We could clearly see what had happened. He had put the 12 gauge shotgun under his chin, and blew all of his brains out through the top of his head.

Unlike the last kid who had tried to end his life with a shotgun, this guy still had a face. The top of his head was gone, and everything inside was spattered across the ceiling.

Then Paul called out, "He still has a heartbeat!" "How can that be?" Rich asked incredulously.

I bent down to check. "Sure enough; he is also breathing," I confirmed. "At least he's trying to breathe."

Apparently even though he had no brain left, the brain stem was still intact. Since the brain stem controls the heart beat and respiration, this explained what seemed impossible. "I'll call the hospital," Paul reported.

"Wait!" Rich called. "If we call, we might have to try to resuscitate him."

"Ok," I agreed, "we'll wait for a few minutes."

Officer Miller walked into the room, followed by another officer I didn't know well. "Do you think there was anything suspicious?" Officer Miller asked.

I shook my head. "Doesn't look like it," I commented.

Officer Miller surveyed the scene and shook his head. "Boy, he really made a mess." We just nodded in silent agreement.

"I talked to the parents," explained Miller. "They said he was depressed. The mother heard the gun shot and called us. She didn't want to see this for herself," said Miller.

A third officer walked in. He was young looking. "This is Officer Donaldson," Miller said to us. "He just started today."

"Welcome to our world," I said sarcastically. Like many new cops, and even new firefighters, this one was gun ho and a bit cocky. I looked at the monitor. The heart was still beating.

"Well, we can't wait any longer," I said. "The doc will probably call it when he finds out what we have."

Rich called the hospital. "Rescue Four to St. Andrews." "St. Andrews here," a nurse answered.

"We have a shotgun wound to the head from under the jaw through the top of his head," Rich reported. "It looks like a suicide. He still has a cardiac rhythm and agonal breathing."

"Standby Rescue Four, I will get the doctor." We waited a few minutes before the doc answered.

"Rescue Four, send me a strip." He meant to send an ECG over the radio. We were expecting that, so it was already ready to send.

"Ok," said the doc, "did you start resuscitation?" "What?" exclaimed Rich.

"Yes!" confirmed the doctor. "Start resuscitation. Start an IV of Ringer's, intubate him and bring him here!"

Bewildered, Rich said, "Ok, we will be there in twenty-five minutes." Paul was already getting the intubation kit and I started the IV. Paul was trying to intubate without much success. "He has no trachea. Or larynx," he pointed out.

I went over to help with the airway. We worked the tube in somehow. While putting the tube in, there were some squeamish noises that I can't even begin to describe. Behind us we heard a burping sound. I looked back and saw the new officer bent over, with his hands over his mouth, yellowish white liquid dripping between his hands. He ran out of the room, and I heard retching from the hallway.

Vomiting is contagious sometimes, and eventually Miller was the only officer left with us. "Where did everyone go?" I teased Miller with a little smile on my face.

"They can't take it, I guess," was his reply.

Just then, the ambulance crew entered the room. "Did you bring your stretcher?" Rich asked them.

"No," admitted the ambulance attendant. "We wanted to see what we had first."

"Now you've seen it," Rich snapped. "Get the stretcher!"

Back then we were having trouble with some of the ambulance crews. The scene was ours, so they were just supposed to bring in the stretcher and transport. But their egos and ours clashed at times. They had to go back out to the ambulance to get the stretcher and bring it back. When they eventually returned, we lifted the body, with an air tube stuck in the skull, onto the stretcher. We let the ambulance crew carry him downstairs and into their vehicle. As we were going down the stairs, Miller asked, "Why did they want you to resuscitate him?"

"I really don't have a good answer for you. I guess since he had a heart rate and was trying to breathe, the Doc thought he had to cover his butt for legal purposes. Maybe he thinks he can harvest his organs. Anyway, we have to comply."

The police stayed behind to investigate the scene while our brainless patient was loaded into the back of the ambulance. I drove the Rescue to the hospital behind it.

The ambulance backed into the stall at the emergency room, and I pulled in next to it. I got out to help move the patient into the emergency room. They now were doing CPR. The ambulance attendants set the stretcher on the cement just outside the ER door. We wheeled him into the room, but there was no nurse or doctor to greet us.

"He went into cardiac arrest just after we left the scene," Paul said as he did chest compressions.

"Here," I said, "let me take over compressions."

There was no argument from Paul, who was grateful for the chance to catch his breath. I stood on the bottom rail of the stretcher while I did chest compressions. The ambulance crew pulled us to an open room, where we parked the stretcher. Doctor Wise, what an ironic name, walked into the room and said, "Time of death 1023," and walked out.

"That's it?" muttered Rich. "All that for what?" Paul and I shared his frustration.

A nurse came into the room and started taking the tubes out and getting the body ready to be taken downstairs to the morgue. We looked at each other in disbelief then took our equipment out to the truck. I put the Rescue back in shape while Rich completed the report.

"I wonder what's going on?" asked Paul when he got back to the Rescue.

"Why?" I asked, uncertain of his meaning.

"This is just a very strange day," he explained. "No one in the ER would even talk to us."

"Well it started out strange enough," I agreed. I will forever have the picture of that boy's head all over the ceiling imprinted in my brain. And that doctor, he was odd, too. We didn't know the strangeness had just begun.

It was about 1100 hours when we got back to the station. It was floor day. The big chore for the day was to strip and wax the kitchen floor. I loved, or should I say, we *all* loved floor day. I'm being sarcastic, of course.

I was hoping the floor would be at least started when we returned. But the two men left back at the station had gone out in the Engine to shop for meals instead. That's ok, I thought. They had a lot of work to do. Bernie was the lieutenant in charge and Bruce was on watch. Bernie said, "We'll do the floors after lunch."

"Sounds good," I said. I looked out at the thermometer, and the temperature outside was 92 degrees. "Ninety-two outside. Good day for a fire," I said with a smile.

"Now you did it!" Paul complained. The guys were so superstitious about that kind of stuff.

"Hot dogs and chips are ready!" Bruce yelled.

"Good, I'm hung--*beeeeeeep*--ry." In mid-sentence, the fire tones went off. Guess I cursed us after all.

"Stations Three and Four, you have a possible suicide at 6793 Camden Place. Time out, 1203."

"What's going on with the suicides?" I protested as we ran to the watch desk. "I've been there before," I said looking at the map. "I was there last week for a domestic. I know right where it is."

Rich took the section map anyway. We ran to the Rescue and climbed in our assigned positions. The apparatus room door was already opening, as I flipped on the lights. We blew the air horn as we pulled out west (right) on Greer. There was no one on the roads.

I turned left, then right onto Willow. We heard, "Engine Three on scene," over the radio.

"Message received, Engine Three."

"Do you know where the house is?" Paul asked from the back.

"Yes," I answered. "Where the big red fire truck is."

We turned left on Keith Road, drove past the ballfields and straight into the subdivision across Commerce Road. There was the red firetruck, lights flashing, in front of a two story house.

"Rescue Four on scene," Rich called in to the mic.

The Engine Three crew had just opened the garage, and smoke poured out the door.

"Don't go in there!" Bob from Engine Three yelled. "The house and garage are filled with carbon monoxide." Engine Three was in the process of setting up the positive pressure fan to force the CO out of the building.

An older man was sitting on the steps of the house. He said sadly, "She's in the car in the in the garage. I don't understand; she seemed so happy."

I approached the man, who was most likely the victim's father, and asked him, "Are you alright? Did you breathe in the carbon monoxide?"

"No," he said, wiping his eyes. "I came over to visit, and when I opened the front door I could smell car fumes. I ran into the garage, and saw her in the car. Then I just went out the side door. I didn't breathe any fumes."

"We should check you out," I said.

"No," the man protested. "I don't want you to touch me. I refuse to let you check me out. I'm fine."

"Ok," I said, "it's your right not to be treated."

He put his hands over his face and simply said, "She's dead." Joe had just come out of the garage with his SCBA on. He took off his mask and said, "No point going in there yet. She's been dead for a long while."

Just then the police arrived. I greeted them as they approached.

"Officer Miller, we meet again. How are you on this crazy day?"

"Going crazy," he replied.

"The garage is clear!" Bob called out. Rich was still trying to get the man to agree to be treated, but he continued to refuse.

We all walked to the garage. There was a white Cadillac in the middle of it. We went up to the car and looked in the window. There was a lady inside, but I couldn't tell much about her condition from there. It was about 120 degrees in the garage.

"Man, it's hot in here," Miller said as he opened the driver's side door. He stuck his head in the car and immediately pulled back.

"It must be three hundred degrees in there!" he exclaimed, rubbing his face where the superheated air had burned it. I looked in the car. What I was looking at did not appear to be human.

"What is that?" Paul echoed my thought when he looked inside.

A body in a red dress was sitting on the driver's side, leaning toward the passenger's side door. Her once-white skin was now brown and tight. You could see the outline of her skull because her skin was so tight. Yellowish fluid dripped from her body onto the seat and car floor. That was melted fat. The odor of burned flesh was strong.

"She's cooked," I stated, still shocked at her condition. "Cooked like a turkey dinner." I repeated. It didn't take long for the car to cool enough for us to see what was going on.

"It doesn't appear that she left a note," Miller reported.

"I can hear a radio," I said. "It's faint, but I hear music."

"The car radio is on," Miller said. "It looks like the engine stalled. The ignition is still on. She might have been listening to music with the car running and the door down when she passed out."

"Then the gas tank must have run dry," I said, pointing out that the engine was currently not operating.

"With the temperature so hot outside and the car running with the door down, it probably made it hot enough that she literally cooked to death," Miller surmised.

Rich looked in briefly before proclaiming, "Yep, she is crispy all right," Rich said, writing on the clipboard for our report.

"Well," Miller said, "what shall I tell the ME; well-done lady?" he muttered as he headed out to his patrol car.

The Engine Three crew had made sure there was no more carbon monoxide in the house, using a CO detector to make sure.

"All clear," Bob pronounced.

"Rescue Four, you can go back."

"Ok, let's go!" I eagerly said, leading the way back to the truck. We stowed the equipment and headed back to our station. Needless to say, the cooked lady was the talk of the ride back.

Rich, with his morbid jokes, kept the others entertained for quite a while when we returned. She was the hot topic of conversation.

"You know, that lady was a really good cook," joked Rich. He especially liked to jest like that at the dinner table. Within a short time, the guys would all be laughing, releasing the stress of the run.

We got through lunch and stripped and waxed the floor without further interruption. We finished all of our chores and sat down in front of the TV to relax.

The next thing I knew, I was startled awake by the sound of, "Dinner is ready!"

"Already? We just had lunch," Paul said rubbing his eyes.

"That was four hours ago!" said the cook. "You remember what our motto is: eat till your tired then sleep till you eat."

"What's for dinner?" I asked. "Roasted hen?" This was met with groans.

After dinner someone asked, "Who wants to play ping pong?" All four of us got up and went downstairs to the ping pong table. I was a pretty good player, but Paul was a master. He was also a master of pool. He would always beat you by one or two points or one ball. In pool, it was always by one ball.

We joked that he had been a pool shark in his past life. He said he could get people to bet money by letting his mark beat him once. Then they would bet money. He would make enough mistakes to beat the mark by one ball. The victim would think he almost won and would bet more thinking he would win next time. The victim always lost by one ball.

Paul would bet on anything. One time he got us to play 'quarters.' We stood ten feet from a wall and we would pitch quarters. Whoever got closest would win all of the thrown coins. Not only was Paul always closest, but his quarters would be leaning against the wall. It didn't take long for us to learn not to bet against him. Today he must have had a bad day because I beat him 21 to 19.

"Do you want to play another game for, let's say five dollars a point?" Paul suggested.

"I don't think so," I replied, knowing his tricks.

Out of nowhere we heard, "Station Four, you have a possible gunshot at the party store at 3999 Hiller Road. Time out, 2230."

"I didn't even hear the tones!" Rich yelled as we scrambled up the stairs and into the watch room. Sometimes down in the basement we wouldn't hear the tones, and it would catch us by surprise. As we reached the watch desk, the lieutenant arrived at the same time.

"We didn't hear the tones," Rich repeated to the lieutenant.

"There weren't any," he replied. Sometimes something would go wrong at dispatch, and they would not send the tones. Then we would be caught off guard. Or we could miss a run.

The lieutenant reached over the desk and keyed the mic and said, "Dispatch, could you please repeat the address?"

"3999 Hiller Road, just north of Greer on the east side of Hiller. Time out, 2231."

We hopped in the Rescue and took off down Greer. "Rescue Four responding," Rich called into the mic.

We quickly arrived at Grove's party store. "Rescue Four on scene. Reporting one man down in the doorway," Rich called into the mic as I pulled the Rescue up to the front of the store.

A man lay on his back at the entrance to the party store, the door half-shut against him. I slammed the Rescue into park, set the parking brakes and ran to the injured man. As we approached, the dispatcher called, "Rescue Four, be advised: do not get out of your truck until the police arrive."

"Too late!" muttered Rich as we reached the victim. The young man, about twenty years of age, was lying on the threshold, half in and half out of the door. Blood was spurting out of his chest.

"What happened?" I yelled to the store manager. He answered as he propped open the door so we could work on the patient.

"He and a neighbor got into an argument. This boy was yelling at another kid. The other one backed him up to the door, pulled out a gun and shot him. It was a .357 Magnum, I think."

"Where is the gunman?" I asked as I looked around.

"He ran out as soon as he shot him."

The hole in the middle of the young man's chest was oozing blood. Rich checked his eyes.

"Fixed and dilated," Rich said. "No pulse." I bandaged the wound quickly.

"Let's go!" Paul called. We all knew that if he had any chance to survive we would have to get him to the hospital ASAP. I noticed a wound in his back.

"The wound is a through and through," I reported. I bandaged that wound as well before we picked up the body and placed it on a backboard. Three police cars arrived, and Officer Miller rushed to help us put him into the Rescue.

Once the patient was secure, Officer Miller asked, "Do you want some help?"

"We could use a hand," I nodded. "Do you think he will survive?"

"Not much chance," I told him as Rich shut the doors.

Though I was supposed to drive, the positions that we ended in dictated where we went. Paul and I were now in the back and Rich was driving. I intubated and bagged the patient while Miller did chest compressions and Paul started the IV line. We hooked up the ECG. It showed a straight line.

"No cardiac activity," Paul stated.

In front, Rich called Sacred Heart Hospital. He relayed their orders to us. "The ER says to give epinephrine and to hurry!"

We looked at each other because we had already given epinephrine, and a few other meds, with no luck. We continued CPR the rest of the way to the hospital. When we backed into the ER stall, we were greeted by three doctors and three nurses. We wheeled the young man into the trauma room.

"How long has he been down?" asked the doctor.

"About ten minutes," I answered.

"Ok," the doctor said, "let's get him on the table."

We stopped CPR while we lifted him to the trauma table. The nurse ripped open the patient's shirt and cleaned his chest with iodine. "Hand me the scalpel," ordered the doctor.

The nurse opened a trauma bag, which held several instruments. She handed the knife to the doctor. He made a long incision over the sternum. Grabbing an instrument out of the trauma kit, the doctor proceeded to cut the sternum open.

"Hand me the spreaders," the surgeon ordered. The nurse slapped the stainless steel spreader in the surgeon's hand. The doctor ripped open the sternum, exposing the patient's organs. His chest cavity was full of blood. The doctor felt around the chest cavity with his gloved hand, feeling his way to the heart. He placed his bloody hand on the heart.

"Shit!" the doctor shouted. "That's it. The heart is shredded. Time of death 2247." A .357 Magnum projectile is so devastating that when it hits tissue it destroys everything around it.

"He never had a chance," the doctor proclaimed. "Good work everyone," he said, snapping off his latex gloves and tossing them in a garbage pail. Everyone watched him as he walked out.

The nurses started to prepare the body for the trip to the morgue, removing all the tubes. I took a peek into his open chest. I could see what was left of the heart in the middle of a pool of partially clotted blood. The cardiac tissue was unrecognizable. It looked to me like a long, flat bunch of reddish string with a large hole in the middle.

I repeated as I walked out, "We did our best, but he did not have a chance." I walked by the nurses' desk and sat beside Paul as he filled out the medical report.

Into the emergency room door came the family of the slain kid. You could always tell the relatives by the way they walked. They were full of fear and uncertainty.

"That must be the family," said Rich, shaking his head.

"Ready to go?"

"I am," said Paul for all of us. "Then let's go home."

As we walked out, we saw the family, a man, woman and girl, probably his sister, disappearing into a counseling room. We put the Rescue back in-service and on the road. It was now 2305 and we were all beat. None of us said anything for quite a while, until Rich spoke up to break the silent downer.

"Well, it sucks to be him."

Paul and I both looked at him and chuckled because only Rich would say something like that.

"I wonder if they caught the shooter?" Paul asked.

"The guy that shot him should be thrown into a wood chipper, feet first, and shot into a cornfield where his shredded remains would be fertilizer. At least then he'd be good for something," Rich suggested with his usual morbidity. That is how Rich got the nickname "Chipper." His answer to dealing with mean or criminal types was to put them into the wood chipper.

We used morbid humor to try to relieve the stress from all the horrific things we saw. None of us would ever admit to being affected by all the death and injuries, but of course we were.

# Chapter 11 - Some Days Duty is Full of Doody

It seemed like I had just shut my eyes and drifted off when the tones roared and the lights crashed on. "Station Four," the dispatcher announced, "you have an infant possibly not breathing at 3564 Huntington Way. We are giving CPR instructions over the phone. Time out, 0711."

That kind of call will wake you up in a hurry; sometimes so fast it hurts. The watchman had already written the address down and was looking it up on the map by the time we reached the watch desk.

Fred, the lieutenant, didn't get out of bed since it was a medical run. Rich grabbed the section map and headed for the rescue. The watchman closed the apparatus room doors after we left, probably heading back to his bunk beside the watch desk. You slept when you could.

"Rescue Four responding," we called to dispatch.

"Responding received, Rescue Four, at 0712 hours." It took about two minutes to get to the address.

"Rescue Four at scene," we called once we were on site.

"Over there," I said, pointing to the side of the road in front of the house. We could see a woman standing there and a man holding an infant.

"Oh no." I knew it wasn't good when they met us at the road.

Rich said, "I'll get in the back. You drive as soon as I tell you I am ready."

Rich took the baby from the father's arms and climbed into the back. The mother scrambled into the front with me.

"My baby! She's not breathing!" she screamed as she closed the door. "How is she doing?" She was frantic.

"We are doing all we can," someone from the back of the truck said. It was a very long ride to the hospital in Pontiac. I really don't want to talk much about the run. All I can say is that it did not turn out well for anyone. Sudden Infant Death Syndrome, known commonly as SIDS, rarely does.

When I got home, my wife, large with our unborn child, was waiting for me. I smiled, thinking that Rich would call that a "whale belly." I pushed thoughts of the recently deceased baby from my head, not wanting to upset Wendy with that tale.

Besides, I had a different problem to deal with just then. Wendy reminded me that I was late for a date with a surgeon. I was supposed to have a large fatty cyst removed from my right forearm. I took a minute to throw some peas and grapes into BeeBe's cage before heading back out the door.

In no time at all, we were off to the doctor's office. Twelve stitches and a few hours later, I was back at home. I spent the rest of the day in bed sleeping and recovering from the surgery.

Wendy and I discussed the imminent birth of our second child, who we knew would be another boy. "Any ideas for a name?" Wendy asked.

"How about Steven Stone?" I suggested. "Or Matthew Robert?"

"I like Matthew Robert." After a pause Wendy added, "What will I do if I go into labor this winter?" We lived in an area that wasn't easily accessible to anything. She was worried about reaching the hospital in time.

"We have cross country skis by the door," I teased.

I liked to go cross country skiing on my days off. I was always exercising and I played many different sports. As a youngster, I remember being the fastest, strongest and biggest kid all the way to high school. I was an all-star baseball player and was a member of the first ever Milford High School varsity ice hockey team. I continued to play softball and hockey until I was about 45 years old. It was a good stress reliever and a fun way to stay in shape.

The night after my surgery, I slept deeply, thankfully without being plagued with weird dreams. Usually, I'd forget most of my dreams as soon as the alarm went off. That was probably a good thing, considering the fodder my brain had at its disposal to create my dreamscapes.

"Time to get up, Gregory!" Wendy yelled to me, waking me from my slumber. It only took me half an hour to get ready for work. That's all the time I had, because I had fallen back to sleep after turning off my alarm. That was unusual for me, but sometimes you just need a little extra.

When I reached Station Three at 0730, the Unit Two cars and Bob's truck were parked in the lot. Although I was half an hour early, I was the last one to get there. When I walked into the living room, Mike immediately asked me to work for him. "I have to take my son to school," he explained.

"No problem," I agreed.

"Thanks!" he said, quickly moving out the door.

Bob and the other Mike were sitting at the round lunch table talking about the house Mike was building.

"The coffee is hot," Bob said to me by way of invitation.

"Good morning men," I said as I reached in the cupboard for a coffee cup. I poured myself a cup of joe and sat down at the table.

Bob said to Mike, "It must be confusing with two Mikes at the same station."

"Not really," Mike disagreed, "we know who we are." There were five Mikes on the fire department and three Johns.

"Hey, did you hear we're getting a new Engine?" Mike said.

"Where did you hear that?" Bob asked him.

"Captain Bill stopped by yesterday and told us that Station One is getting a new pumper, and we will get the old Engine One."

"It will be nice to have an automatic instead of a double-clutching stick," I said after I took a sip of coffee.

Mike got up from the table and announced, "Well, I've got places to go and people to do." He was always mixing up phrases for our entertainment. "See you tomorrow?" he asked me.

I replied, "Will you be here in the morning?"

"Yes, I will. See you in the morning."

With that, he walked out the door. Bob and I watched the news and drank coffee until 0815.

"Well," I said, getting up from the table, "I'll go check out my truck."

I walked out to the apparatus room to inspect the three vehicles. The first was Engine Three, followed by Tanker Three, which holds two thousand gallons of water. The last to get my attention was the pickup. We always kept a first aid and IV kit in that truck.

It took about an hour to complete the task. When I was finished, I went to the watch room. Bob had more seniority than me, and with no lieutenant today, he was in charge, leaving me on watch. The watch room was a tiny place, only about five by twelve feet. The desk took up half of that space.

Bob was finished with the log and his blue in-charge slip, which had to be filled out in order to allow him to get paid about a dollar an hour more for the day. He was now busy doing crossword puzzles.

Part of being on watch duty meant you had to do the grocery shopping and cooking. I had just pulled into the Kroger parking lot, opened the door and stepped one leg out when I heard dispatch on the radio.

"Station Three and Rescue Four, you have a medical emergency, a possible drug overdose at 77886 Dandison, located behind Station Three. Time out, 0920."

I pulled my leg back into the truck, shut the door and picked up the mic, saying, "Utility Three responding."
As I pulled out of the parking lot, I turned on my emergency lights and sped east on Commerce Road.

"Engine Three enroute."

"Enroute received, Engine Three, at 0921."

It only took me a minute to get to the scene. Engine Three got there almost immediately. Dandison was right behind their station, west of Green Lake Road.

"Utility on scene," I said, opening the door and running down the pitted sidewalk to an old, run-down house.

I opened the front door just in time to see Bob being lifted up into the air by a scrawny 110 pound, five foot tall druggie. The guy's eyes were wide open, bloodshot and crazy.

He yelled, "Get the hell out of my house!" as he threw a screaming Bob across the room. Bob crash-landed on a tattered brown couch that was covered with black stains and cigarette burns. His momentum flipped the couch over, dumping him on the floor between the upside-down couch and a peeling, once-white wall. Bob just lay there for a moment, dazed.

Two police officers came in the door, one of them our friend Officer Miller. Without saying a word, all three of us rushed the full-body tattooed drug addict. The other officer, who probably weighed three hundred pounds, grabbed the guy's arm.

"Get off me!" Druggie screamed, slamming the large officer into a dirty wall. He slid, stunned, down the wall onto his butt. He briefly shook his head and then got back up. Bob had re-joined the struggle, followed by the officer who'd been knocked down. All four of us grabbed Druggie at once.

"I'm going to kill you!" Druggie screamed again as he fought us. Bob grabbed his left arm, Miller took the right and the other cop and I took the body. We tackled the crazed man to the floor.

"Settle down!" Miller yelled as he slapped handcuffs on one wrist. The patient grabbed my forearm and squeezed tightly, pulling me to him and falling on top of me.

The free handcuff whistled past my head and slammed to the floor. Two more officers had arrived and pulled the guy off me. Between the six of us, we slapped the cuffs on him as he lay face down on the floor, four officers pinning him down. He still struggled to get up, screaming constantly and incoherently.

Druggie's sister arrived and burst into the house. "Don't hurt him!" she screamed.

"What is he on?" I asked her.

"He is on meth and I don't know what else," she replied.

The ambulance crew entered the house with the stretcher. Rescue Four's crew also came into the room. We lifted the struggling man onto the stretcher and strapped his arms and body down.

"Sorry we were delayed," Tom from Rescue Four said, trying to explain. I couldn't focus on what he said with all the confusion and honestly, I really didn't care. I needed to stay attentive to my job.

"What's he on?" asked Tom.

"I have been kind of busy, Tom," I replied. "The only thing that I know is he on is meth and some other unknown substance."

"Did you check his room?" Tom asked.

"No, I was busy fighting with the patient!" I snapped impatiently.

"You have blood on your arm," Tom told me.

I looked down. Sure enough blood was dripping off my forearm. A closer look told me that all of the stitches from my recent surgery had popped open. "Great!" I muttered as I went to the trauma box.

I was dressing my wound when Tom announced, "We didn't find any more drugs. We will take over here."
To me he said, "You'd better go get that checked out."

"I will," I said, but I knew that I wouldn't, at least not until tomorrow after work. I watched Rescue Four and the ambulance as they wheeled the crazed man out the door, with his sister following and giving orders.

Officer Miller came up to me and asked, "How can such a tiny, scrawny man be so strong? He threw Officer Murphy against the wall! It took six of us to get him under control. Unbelievable!"

"Yeah," I agreed, "he also threw Bob across the room. He crashed right into that couch."

Some drugs, like meth, or a mixture of different uppers, will make a person delusional. Epinephrine is released into the bloodstream in large amounts, giving the user great strength.

"Hey, what happened to your arm?" Officer Miller asked as he noticed the bandage.

"Oh, he popped my stitches when we were fighting with him. He got a hold of my arm," I answered.

"You should go to the hospital," Miller told me.

"I will," I assured him, looking to close the subject.

"Bob, are you ok?" I asked. "It's a good thing that you landed on that couch."

"I'm fine," Bob said.

"What's that on your knees?" I asked as I examined his pants.

Then I realized what it was.

"It's dog poop!" I told him.

"What?" Bob screeched. He was squeamish about things like that. "I thought I smelled dog shit!" he added.

He started laughing and pointed to my pants, saying, "You've got dog shit all over your pants too!"

I looked down. Sure enough, Bob was right. "You'd better change your shirt too," he added, pointing to the blood smeared on my uniform.

"Crap!" I said as Bob started laughing again. "Literally!" We picked our way across the room toward the front door, avoiding the scattered land mines on the floor. Miller met us at the door and dropped the bombshell.

"There are no dogs here."

Back at the station, we showered and put on new uniforms. We all keep an extra set of clothes in our locker for emergencies just like this. We threw our poopy clothes in the ancient washing machine. That thing was so old it still had a clothes wringer attached.

We had just arrived back in the living room when the phone rang. Bob answered it, looking over at me while he was talking and said, "Ok, Chief. I will tell him."

When he hung up the phone, he said, "The Chief wants you to take the utility truck and go to Henry Ford Hospital to get that arm fixed *now*!" He added, "Maybe if you play it right, you can get the rest of the week off."

"I'll do my best," I agreed. "The Chief said to go to Ford, so to Ford I will go."

Fire Department policy said we were supposed to go to the hospital if we got injured, no matter how minor. The Department pays for it, so it's not a big deal.

As I was walking out the door, Bob said, "I will do your injury report."

"Thanks, Bob." We always had to fill out an injury report and record it in the log, no matter how small the incident.

After about four and a half hours in the waiting room, I was finally brought to an examination room. After about another hour, the doctor came in. The first thing he said to me was, "You smell like shit!"

Apparently the shower did not get rid of the smell. The doctor struggled to ignore the rank odor as he sewed up my arm. He ordered me to take the rest of the day off. "I can do that," I agreed, happily. As I was driving home I thought, "No wonder no one would sit by me in the waiting room." I wouldn't sit next to someone who reeked of shit either!

I called my wife to warn her I was coming home early. She met me at the door and leaned in to kiss me. The stench hit her and she quickly pulled back, saying, "You stink!"

As it turned out, I still got the week off, because Wendy went into labor at five in the afternoon that same day. We had a new baby boy, Matthew Robert Johnson. There's nothing like seeing your own son being born.

Matthew was a ten on the Apgar scale. Nothing wrong with that kid's lungs. After we took him home, we didn't get much sleep for quite a while. There is an old tongue-in-cheek saying in the Fire Department,

"Having a baby won't change my life." That saying started when a young father-to-be said that, and believed it. He, like every new parent, found out he was wrong.

# Chapter 12 - General Hospital; Detroit Style

In addition to being into sports, I was in marching band and concert band through high school. My mom had been an art teacher, and I went to Central Michigan University for music, planning to become a teacher as well. Fortunately, I realized early on that I wasn't cut out for that career, and instead decided to go into the new field of emergency medicine. I attended Wayne State for my basic EMT license and then Madonna University for advanced EMT.

When I hired in at WBFD, I was one of the first employees with EMT training. Like other professions, we were expected to put in a certain number of hours of training to maintain our license. And of course, the Department paid fees to keep things current as well.

The next day, I received a call from Station One informing me that I had to go to Detroit General Hospital to do rotations to earn points for my medic license. I was expected to go on my only day off. Between the marionette shows and the Fire Department, I didn't get much time off, but at least I got overtime pay.

The next day, as I drove to Detroit General, I realized how much I hated rotations. Not much good would happen at General. I had two rotations to complete in eight hours. First was psychiatric. The second would be in the emergency room. It was difficult to say which was worse.

For the first rotation at 0700 hours, I met Dr. Schmart at his office. He walked in at 0705 and we talked about what we would see. "Just remember," he warned me, "don't wear your stethoscope around your neck. The patients may grab it and try to choke you."

I could tell that he was annoyed that he had to have me around. He brought me outside his office. The ER was crowded and there were stretchers with patients lining the halls, most of them crazy and strapped down. There would be screaming and people talking to no one. It was unsettling at best. He gave orders to the nurse,

"Send in the first patient."

"Yes, Dr. Schmart," said the nurse.

We walked back to his office and waited for the patient to arrive. He warned me, "Don't say anything while I am consulting, ok?"

"I won't," I promised. The nurse opened the office door and announced, "Here is Mr. Smith."

Mr. Smith walked in and sat down. The nurse closed the door. I don't remember exactly what the doctor asked, but it immediately set the patient off. I think he asked him his name. I could see the patient was getting agitated.

His face got tight and all of a sudden he bolted out of his chair right towards the doctor. I saw the doctor's look of terror for a split second. I didn't have any time to think. I just reacted, feeling like I was watching from somewhere else.

Leaping out of my chair, I tackled the guy, slamming him to the floor. He was much bigger than me, so I was glad the two huge orderlies ran in and subdued him. Then they took him away. Dr. Schmart was visibly shaken.

"Thank you for taking him down," he said to me.

"I just reacted before I knew what was happening," I answered. "I've had that happen once before, and the EMT didn't even move," Dr. Schmart told me. "Lucky for me he was a slow man, and the orderly got to me in time to stop him," he continued. "This patient, however, could have killed me."

"He was big and fast," I agreed. Then I added, half-jokingly, "It was fun!" In a more serious tone, I admitted, "But I did react before I knew what I was getting in to. If I would have had time to think about it, I would have realized I could have been hurt, or sued. It worked out, though, right?"

Dr. Schmart was regaining his composure. "Ok," he said with a quiver in his voice, "we are done for the day. I will fill out your report and give you credit for four hours. Thanks again," he added. "Come on, I'll buy you some breakfast."

We went down to the cafeteria and had a nice breakfast and a good talk. After, Dr. Schmart made some calls so I wouldn't have to wait around for hours for my next rotation.

"You can start your next rotation in the ER now, if you want," he told me.

"I think I will," I replied. "Thank you, Dr. Schmart."

He led me to the ER, said good bye and wished me luck. Then he turned and walked away, disappearing around the corner. I had taken only one step when I felt a tug on my neck. I was forcefully pulled onto a stretcher, my neck being choked by my own stethoscope. I started to become light-headed when the same two orderlies pulled me away from the patient that had grabbed me.

The orderlies both said, "Didn't anybody tell you not to wear your stethoscope around your neck?" at the same time. "It could be dangerous!" they added.

All I could say was "thanks," as I rubbed my neck, feeling like an idiot. It shows to go you, you can be up one minute and down the next. Needless to say, I never wore my stethoscope around my neck there again.

The rooms and halls were overcrowded in that place. Worse, most of the patients were as crazy as I've ever seen. They tried to grab me and everyone else passing by. They yelled and screamed. A big woman was standing at the nurses' desk, yelling that she was having chest pain. In the confusion, no one took notice of her until she collapsed to the floor. I was close to her, so I was the first to reach her. I was immediately knocked away by the big orderlies.

"Code Blue at nurses' station," came over the loudspeaker. Nurses rushed up to the lady with a stretcher. We all helped lift her onto the cot as CPR was started. She was whisked away into a nearby room. Until that moment, I hadn't realized that she had emptied her bowels onto the floor…and my shoes.

I just stood there, dumbfounded. I blankly glanced toward the room where the woman had been taken. I wondered, "What just happened?"

By the time I cleaned my shoes, things had slowed down a bit. Finally, the nurse that was supposed to show me around arrived. She was about to tell me what was expected of me when an announcement came in. A triple shooting involving a police officer was arriving in a few minutes.

I followed the nurse to the ER door just as Detroit EMS arrived. Two doctors, three nurses and I met the ambulance. Lying on the stretcher as we wheeled him into the ER was a young police officer. He looked no older than about twenty-five. His whole head was bandaged up, and blood was seeping through the gauze on the left side of his head. I was handed the IV bag as we pushed the young officer into trauma room four.

One of the EMTs said, "He is stable, breathing on his own. His BP is 140/70. There are two more on the way."

"What is their condition?" asked one doctor.

"One officer has a leg wound, and a minster has been shot in the forehead. I don't think he will make it. The shooter is dead. They should be here in about two minutes."

"We will need another trauma team in room two," a doctor ordered. A nurse left to organize the second team. The rest of us worked on the young patient.

"Give me an x-ray stat!" another doctor ordered. The technician was already there, getting the portable machine ready.

Meanwhile, we checked over the patient. He was moaning, but not conscious. A doctor did neurologic tests to find out if the officer had any brain injuries. "Everything seems normal," he announced after checking the patient's feet for reflexes. The x-ray technician said, "I am ready to take pictures."

"Everyone out!" the doctor ordered.

We filed out to let the tech do his job. The doctors didn't want to take the bandages off until they saw what they had. The x-ray showed that the projectile had entered the officer's left eye area before fragmenting into three large pieces and a lot of smaller pieces.

"Ok, let's get him up to surgery," one of the doctors ordered.

A nurse told him, "The OR team is scrubbing. They will be ready in about fifteen."

"The sooner the better, because his brain is showing signs of swelling." After a pause, the doctor added, "We'd better get him intubated. We will do a tracheotomy in the OR."

The nurses cut through the bandages to get to his mouth. The bandage came off long enough to get to the airway. In that moment, I saw the wound. His left eye was gone. Blood was oozing out of the hole where his eye used to be. He moaned as the bandages were replaced. "He is regaining consciousness," a nurse said.

The doctor ordered a drug given through the IV to allow the endotracheal tube to be inserted. An anesthesiologist was at the head of the patient, ready to put in the airway.

"Here," he motioned to me, "put in the tube."

I took the tube and laryngoscope. I was good at intubating, so it didn't take me long. When I finished, it was time to take him up to surgery. As the officer was being wheeled to the elevator, more patients entered the ER.

The next one in was an elderly black pastor of a local church. He had blood oozing out of a hole in his forehead. He already had a tube in and was being bagged because he was not breathing on his own.

"His BP is 240/190, the heart rate 180 BPM," the medic rattled off to whoever would listen. The patient also had an IV started.

Right behind him was another police officer lying on a stretcher with his right thigh bandaged. "This one is stable," a medic said, indicating the officer.

"Put him in room one," a nurse ordered, "and put the reverend in five. You," she pointed to me, "go into five with him and help out there."

I helped push the patient into room five. Just then Detroit police officers were beginning to arrive. I took over the bag mask and began bagging the reverend. The respiratory therapist was already there to hook him up to a breathing machine that would breathe for him. It didn't take her long to set up the machine and attach him to it. With every "shhhhh" noise, I could see his chest rising. We got an x-ray for him, but the doctor said there was nothing we could do to help him. I was told to stay there and watch him for a while.

A short time later, I noticed something gray, with blood on it, coming out of his nose. I leaned in to look more closely when a big glob of gray matter blew out of his left nostril and onto the floor with a splat. "That is part of his brain," a voice from behind me said exactly what I had been thinking. I looked back at the nurse who was in charge of me for the day.

"His brain swelled so much from the trauma that the brain tissue was squeezed out." She added, "The officer that shot the suspect told me that he was called to the scene for a domestic dispute. Reverend Jones here was walking up the steps to talk to the shooter, try to reason with him and talk him down. The suspect had been pointing a gun at his girlfriend, but suddenly turned the gun on the reverend and shot him first, then the police officer. That's when the other officer shot the suspect." She paused. "The officer with the head wound should be ok, but he lost his eye. At least his other eye is fine."

"Good," I replied. Suddenly, the Reverend went into cardiac arrest. The monitor was screaming as he went into V-fib. I hurried to help him.

"Just let him go," the nurse said quietly, walking over to him and covering his head with a sheet. She could tell he was beyond help.

What a day, and technically it had just started. The time went by quickly. There were a half dozen minor gunshot wounds and a few DOAs and a lot of psych and overdose patients. Nothing, however, compared to that first hour.

I have to admit that what I witnessed bothered me for a long while. There's nothing like seeing a young family crowded around a gravely wounded father that was just trying to do his job. When my hospital rotation was over, I was exhausted. I got home, just wanting to fall into bed. It was not to be, however, because I had a new baby son and my toddler to deal with. Sleep was a sacrifice I was willing to make in exchange for being a father. It brought some normalcy into my life.

# Chapter 13 - Man's Best Friend

I opened the door to Station Four and was greeted by the station officer, Lt. Bigger. He was a skinny guy, about 5'10" and balding, with a good sense of humor. "Chief wants you to call him ASAP."

"Ok, thanks John." I called the lieutenant John rather than by his title, because we came up through the ranks together. In fact, I actually had more seniority than him. Only four medics had been in the department longer than me. He had chosen to rank up in his career, whereas I hadn't. I had a family and a business to run, so I didn't have time to study for the officer's test. It wasn't a priority for me.

I jokingly asked John, "What did I do now?" He shrugged with a smile. Guess I'd have to find out for myself. The phone rang on the other end briefly before it was answered.

"Chief's Office, Chief Borg speaking." Chief Benson had retired and Borg took over.

"Hi Carl, it's Greg. You wanted me to call you?" The new chief and I were also on a first name basis, because we had been friends before he was promoted.

"We need a paramedic at Station Four because Bruce is out with an injury. Would that cause a problem with your business?" Before I could respond, he added, "It wouldn't change your Kelly."

The chief technically did not have to ask if it would be alright with me or if it would affect my business, but that was the kind of man he was. "Thanks for asking, Chief. No, it wouldn't bother my business. When would I be transferred?" I asked.

"How about today?" he responded. "I will have your paper work out with the station mail."

"Sounds good, Chief."

"Have a safe day, Greg." I hung up the phone and turned to the rest of the guys. "Well," I announced, "today is your lucky day! I'm being transferred."

John asked, "Where to?"

"Here. Permanently!" Everyone said at once, "Oh no!" They were joking of course, or at least I think they were.

I walked into the kitchen to get a cup of coffee and there, eating yesterday's leftovers, was a big, skinny black lab. "Who is this?" I asked, bending down to ruffle the dog's ears in a friendly greeting.

"His name is Bugsy," answered John. "He lives across the field in the log house."

My eyebrows raised in surprise. "You mean that the people who were hitting golf balls at our cars own him?"

"That's them," John agreed as he petted the big dog.

"Fred from Unit Two has been feeding him. Now the damn dog won't leave."

"Why should he?" asked Ray II, not to be confused with my friend Rusty-Ray.

As I petted Bugsy, he looked at me with big brown eyes. I was a sucker for animals and animals seemed to know it. "Sounds good to me," I said, knowing I had made a new friend.

"Finish your joe, we have the floors to do," John ordered.

One of the worst chores was washing the apparatus room floors with oil soap twice a week. I chugged the rest of my coffee and filed out with the others. The first one into the room pushed the "all doors up" button. After we checked the trucks, it was time to wash the floors. Ray II was already there throwing a tennis ball against the wall.

Bugsy chased the ball as it bounced around the slippery smooth floors. The ball hit the wall and bounced back. The dog slid into the wall, his legs still running. It took about five seconds before he could stop the forward motion and turn the other way. It looked hilarious. We all laughed and took turns throwing the ball against the walls to watch Bugsy crash, slip and slide all over the floor. No one enjoyed it more than Bugsy. He loved it!

Eventually, we had to get to work. I took the mop bucket to the back room where we kept the soap. The oil soap was in a 55 gallon barrel. I had to lift off the metal top and scoop two full shovels of condensed soap into the bucket. Then, I'd go over to the slop sink and pour hot water with a hose into the bucket and mix it up. As I was filling the bucket, the others were using other hoses to wet the floor. That made the floor slippery, but not as slippery as when we put soap down.

We all grabbed a mop and dunked them in the soapy water and slapped them to the floor. The four of us spread the soap until the whole floor was covered.

Bugsy dropped the tennis ball on my foot. I picked up the ball and meant to throw it out the apparatus room door. The big black dog ran towards the open door, but the ball hit the column between the doors and bounced back. Bugsy tried to stop but skidded right out the door. "That was funny," said Ray as he picked the ball up.

Bugsy ran back in and sat in front of Ray, waiting with his mouth wide open, staring at the ball. Ray threw the ball at the side wall, bouncing it on an angle to the front wall and back to us. Bugsy tried to follow the ball but his feet slipped as he started to run. He was running as fast as he could, but he didn't go anywhere. Finally, his feet were no longer under him and he fell on his belly with his legs spread in all four directions.

Everyone thought that was so funny, and we kept throwing the ball and watching Bugsy having great fun sliding across the floor and crashing into the wall. He always came back for more. Finally, he got hot and tired. That dog was so smart. He had noticed where the water came from in the slop sink on the floor. He trotted over to it and stepped in, waiting to be hosed down. We rinsed the soap off Bugsy and the floor. The wet, happy dog took the ball and laid out on the grass in the sun for a short rest.

After we rinsed off the floor, we took the squeegees and pushed the water into the grates set into the floors. With everything bright and clean, we headed to the door leading back into the living quarters, Bugsy following right behind. As the door opened, Bugsy pushed his way in first and ran into the kitchen to finish his leftovers.

We poured ourselves another cup of joe, then sat around the lunch table for a break.

Unfortunately for us, dog plus greasy leftovers equals bad dog gas. Nothing smells quite like dog fumes. Boy could that dog could fart. Firefighters pride themselves on their farts, in case you didn't know. Some guys could fart on command. Sometimes farts were graded on tone quality, volume, length and most importantly, smell. After the meals we ate, we had some really great contests. Bugsy could fart with the best of us.

I used the brick wall behind the station to bounce a ball off to warm up for my softball games or just for exercise. I used a super ball so it would come back fast. I got my glove and ball out of my car.

Somehow, Bugsy knew that I had a ball in my glove and sat in front of me waiting impatiently. Standing about forty feet from the wall, I threw the ball, aiming to hit about halfway up. Bugsy chased it on its way in, but then it rebounded off the pavement and into the air over his head back to me.

He stopped and jumped way up into the air, just missing the ball as I caught it. But he never missed again, if it was within his reach. The wall stood about five feet high. As good of a shot as I was, I sometimes overthrew it and watched it sail over the top. That was a problem because the other side of the wall was overgrown with thick brush, weeds and thorny plants. Usually, I would just get out another ball, unless it was my last one.

This time when I threw the ball over the wall, I thought I was done for the day. Then Bugsy went after it. Almost effortlessly, he leapt over the wall and then quickly jumped back over, the ball in his mouth. He bounded over and dropped it at my feet. I played catch with that silly dog until he got too hot. Then he ran into the apparatus room and sat in the slop sink, waiting to be hosed off. With that dog hanging around, I could finally play catch with someone.

I had already asked Rusty-Ray to cover me that night so I could go to my softball game. Always dependable, he arrived at 1600 hours. "Thanks for coming in for me, Rusty-Ray."

"No problem, Gregory."

"You'll be driving the Rescue," I called to him as I walked to my truck. I was looking forward to my ball game, thinking about strategies to defeat our next opponent as I drove towards the field. Then something shiny came into view on Newton Road, right in front of Multi-Lakes Sports Club. As I got a little closer, I could see it was a motorcycle, lying in the middle of the road, with smoke pouring up from it.

"That's strange," I thought to myself as I stopped the truck. There was no one around. I knew there had to be someone injured around there. The bike didn't crash itself.

I decided to look around. To my left, in a ditch beside the driveway, was a black jacket. I pulled into the Multi-Lakes driveway and saw the rider in the ditch. I grabbed my first-aid kit from the back of my truck and ran to him.

The guy was moaning, and I could see at a glance he had two open fractures of his tibia and fibula. The bones in both lower legs were tearing out of his pants. He also had a right fractured humerus, a left radius fracture and a fractured ulna.

"Help me!" the injured man cried when he saw me.

"I'm here," I tried to console him. "I'm a paramedic. Help will be coming soon."

A car stopped next to us. Without hesitation I yelled, "Call 9-1-1!" Then I went back to work.

"Are you having any trouble breathing?"

"No," he answered.

"I'm going to bandage your legs," I told him.

He said to me, "My legs don't feel so good."

"Yeah, I'm afraid they are broken," I answered calmly. "My arms are too?" the injured man asked.

"Yes they are, but help is coming."

I bandaged the open wounds, but I couldn't do much else without splints. So, I stayed with him for comfort. It took about eight minutes before I heard sirens. This was not West Bloomfield territory, but rather Commerce's. They had a good department, but at that time it was mostly volunteers, which would take a little longer because volunteers had to come from home to the station first to get the trucks. Then they had to drive to the scene.

I was still kneeling beside the rider when Commerce Township Fire Department came on the scene. A few minutes later, the ambulance arrived, followed by the Oakland County Sheriffs. I gave the officer and the Commerce crew a quick review of what I had learned.

"I am a firefighter paramedic at West Bloomfield. He was struck by a hit and run car while pulling out of Multi-Lakes. His legs have open fractures, and he has upper arm and lower arm fractures. His airway is good."

"Thanks," said the head firefighter, "we will take over now." "He will need a backboard," I reminded him.

"I know!" he said curtly, as eight firefighters and the ambulance crew swarmed the patient. I got up and went to my car. I headed back on the road towards my game. I was thinking to myself that they hadn't asked me my name, which was good. That way I didn't have to worry about being sued or get into any trouble for trying to help someone.

"Oh well!" I thought. "That took up forty-five minutes. Maybe I can get in one or two innings at least."

However, as I pulled into the softball field parking lot, I could see the players walking back to their cars. The manager came up to my car. "Where have you been?" he complained. "We lost because of you!"

This was before cell phones were common, so I hadn't been able to call and let them know why I was late. "Sorry. I stopped at a motorcycle accident. The rider was really messed up," I explained.

"Well, see you next week, right?"

"Sounds good," I replied. As I drove back to the station, I thought, "I stop at an accident, miss a ballgame, waste a trade and lose the game." Not the best kind of night.

When I reached the Station Four parking lot, there was Bugsy waiting for me. He had become very fond of me, probably because I would play with him. I had also became fond of him. He was a good friend.

"Thanks, Rusty-Ray," I said as I entered the kitchen area. The men had just finished dinner and were in the process of cleaning up. Rusty-Ray was just walking out the door as the tones went off.

"Station Four, Rescue Four you have a possible shooting at 7577 Apple Berry Road. Time out, 2122."

Lt. Bigger announced, "We'll take the Engine and Rescue." We filed out the door as Lt. Bigger pulled out the section map. He pushed the door up button and hopped in the passenger side of the Engine, while Bruce jumped into the driver's seat. Meanwhile, I pulled out the Rescue with Ray II sitting in shotgun.

"Engine Four and Rescue Four are responding," Lt. John said over the radio.

"Engine Four and Rescue Four responding received, Engine Four. Be advised Apple Berry runs north off of Willow Road." The dispatcher continued the message, "Also stage at Willow and Apple Berry until the police arrive."

"Message received, dispatch."

We pulled behind the Engine, with lights and siren blaring, onto Greer Road. We turned right on Hiller then right again onto Willow. Just before we reached Apple Berry, we turned off our lights so as not to be a target or to upset anything going down.

"Dispatch, Engine Four and Rescue Four staging at Willow and Apple Berry," Lt. Bigger radioed as we came to a stop at the side of the road.

"Message received. Be advised the police will be there in about two minutes," the dispatcher said. When we pulled to the side of the road, dust and gravel were kicked up by the tires. It hung like a shroud around the trucks for a short time. Staging means that we must wait at a designated area until told differently. You can stage at an assigned area on a fire if you are not needed yet. Or, like in our case, if there is a possible threat.

I could see a flashing blue light in the distance, followed shortly thereafter by the wail of a police siren. The blue lights were getting closer until the patrol car flew past as he flashed his spotlight at us. The sedan slid on the turn a little and kicked up gravel and dust. I could hear the gravel bouncing off the side of the Rescue.

A few minutes later, the dispatcher came over the radio, "Engine Four, you can proceed to the scene. Police reporting one man down with gunshot wound and the shooter is in custody."

"Message received," the lieutenant replied. We continued to the scene. As we arrived, two more patrol cars pulled up. The new officers ran out and disappeared behind the house.

"Engine Four and Rescue Four on scene," called Lt. Bigger.

"Message received, Engine Four."

We stopped the trucks and I went around to the side of the Res- cue to help get the equipment. Bruce handed me the LIFEPAK and the oxygen. I turned around as Bruce jumped out of the side door. We started running towards the dark house. The only lights we could see were the flashlight beams from the police officers darting around. We heard a voice.

"Over here!" It came from the flashlight on the other side of the house. A beam of light shone into my face as the officer's voice said again, "Over here! A man down over here."

We ran towards the flashlight. I stumbled and slipped on the uneven ground as we got closer. There was dew on the grass, soaking through my shoes. We finally reached the officer.

"This way," he said, leading us to the back of the house. A bright patio light was shining on the back porch, so we could see a little better. There was a long dark form lying on the grass about twenty five feet from the porch.

The officer led us up to the patient, telling us that he was a process server who had been trying to serve a subpoena. "He'd been trying to serve this subpoena for a long time and had finally caught up to the suspect."

Apparently, the suspect wouldn't answer the door, but the server kept trying to get it to the suspect, bugging him until he lost his temper. The suspect then snuck up behind the server and shot him in the back. The police had the accused in custody, at least.

As the officer finished giving us the information, we reached the wounded patient. He was a large man of about forty years old. He was moaning, lying face down. He had blood coming out of his back, just below his lungs and to the right of his spine. The bullet appeared to have missed his spine by about an inch and a half. All four of us knelt beside him. "Can you hear me?" I asked as I leaned close to his head to listen to his breathing.

"I hear you," he answered, "but I can't move my legs. He shot me in the back!" He said this with surprise in his voice. "I still served him the subpoena."

"Do you have any trouble breathing?" I asked.

"No. I can breathe just fine, but I can't move my f'ing legs!" The patient followed this by asking, "Did they catch that son of a bitch?"

"Yes. they caught him," I answered; glad I could at least give him that satisfaction. "Let's not worry about that now," I continued, "we've got to get you to the hospital."

"I can't believe that son of a bitch f'ing shot me!" This guy was pissed, and I couldn't blame him, either. He didn't know it yet, and neither did I, but his life would be changed forever.

I ripped opened his shirt to expose the wound. The officer shone his light on it so we could see. It was a very small hole in his back, with some blood oozing out. "What type of gun was used? Do you know?" I asked the officer that had the flashlight.

He said, "It was a .22 revolver." That explained the small wound, I thought to myself. There was not much blood coming from it, but that didn't mean much. He could still bleed out internally and we wouldn't see it. Usually, gunshot wounds, especially from close range, are through and through wounds, meaning the bullet passes through the body. But in this case, when I checked his front side for an exit wound there was none.

"No exit wound," I announced, as I finished running my hand under the front of his body. We couldn't turn him over to check for exit wounds because that movement could cause permanent paralysis. We bandaged him and took his blood pressure. It was 150/100. I listened to his lungs, which sounded clear, and started an IV line. I couldn't get his respirations because he would not shut up. He issued a stream of complaints and threats.

"That son of a pup shot me. I will get that f'er!" It went on and on. Since he had the strength to keep up the tirade, I guess his breathing was good enough.

Lt. Bigger had gone back to the Rescue and picked up the long backboard. We set the board beside him, and all four of us lifted him carefully onto it. He was screaming in pain as we moved him.

Ray said to him, "We will get you something for the pain when we get you to the ambulance."

Lt. Bigger took the hand radio and said, "Dispatch, can you get a twenty on the ambulance?"

"Ok, Engine Four, stand by." A *twenty* was from the old ten code we used to use. It meant "give me a location."

The dispatcher came back shortly and said, "The ambulance should be on the scene." Just as she finished her transmission, the ambulance crew showed up with their stretcher. All six of us lifted him onto it.

The Engine and Rescue had their bright spot lights on, illuminating the way so we could see and not stumble on the way back to the ambulance. After we put the patient in the ambulance, we gave him some morphine. Needless to say, he became a lot happier.

I followed the ambulance in the Rescue all the way to the hospital. Ray II and Bruce had accompanied the patient. Lt. Bigger took Engine Four back to the station by himself. It was an uneventful ride. When we arrived at the hospital, there was no one to greet us at the door and there was no place to park. The ER was packed.

I parked the Rescue on the driveway beside another Rescue from Pontiac Fire Department. That department no longer even exists. I went over to the ambulance, and they already had the patient out. I helped wheel him into the ER. The place was hopping. Doctors and nurses were scurrying around with clipboards. We stopped for a moment and looked around, hoping someone would notice us.

"It must be a Saturday night," Ray II said.

Finally, a triage nurse came up to us and said, "This must be our gunshot patient."

"Correct ma'am," Ray II answered. She led us into a trauma room that had another patient.

"It's kind of crowded tonight," she said, stating the obvious. "I will get a doctor." To my surprise, it didn't take very long before one came in with a nurse. We gave him the report, and he went to the head of the patient and said, "You've had a rough day, I see."

"You can say that again," the patient answered.

"Well, let me check you out." The doctor went to his feet and took a pen out of his pocket. He rubbed it against the bottom of his foot and asked, "Can you feel this?"

The patient answered, "No."

I felt bad for the man. It was not a good sign that he couldn't feel what the doctor was doing. After the examination, the doctor ordered x-rays. I helped Ray II do the medical report at the nurses' station. Then I went back to the patient's room and looked at the x-rays. I could see that the bullet had passed near the spine, but missed it. However, fragments of the bullet had bounced around and lodged in a few different places in his abdomen.

I've heard people say that because a .22 is a small, low-velocity bullet, it doesn't cause much damage. In reality, while it does not cause the tissue damage like a high-velocity round does, it bounces around inside the body and off of bones, often causing great damage. But I could see in the x-ray that the bullet had missed the spine. Maybe the feeling would come back to his legs.

The doctor came into the room and saw me looking at the x-rays. "What do you see?" he asked. I told him what I noticed and what I thought it meant. "Yes, you're right, but he'll be going up for surgery in a few minutes."

"He'll be able to walk again, right?" I asked.

"Not likely," the doctor shook his head. "There is too much swelling, which might have permanently injured the spinal cord." Seeing my expression, I think the doctor felt bad about his blunt assessment. "But, time will tell," he added, more gently. "I have to get back to work," he told me and then walked out.

My heart sank. I felt bad for the patient. I had thought he would recover, but I was wrong.

On the way back to the station, I was thinking of all the things that I'd seen destroy peoples' lives. The young people that were killed in car and motorcycle accidents, toddlers run over, crib deaths, the murder of a young man, and now this senseless shooting, leaving a man paralyzed for the rest of his life. It wasn't only the thought of the people who were injured or killed.

Having a family of my own, I couldn't even imagine what it would feel like if I lost a child. Back in those days, the Fire Department didn't offer counseling for fire and rescue personnel. We were left to deal with it in our own way.

It was nice to see Bugsy's smiling furry face waiting for us when we reached Station Four. Bugsy was smart enough to stay out of the way when the trucks left on runs or returned to the station, but he always happily greeted us once it was safe.

The dog followed us into the bunk room, seeming to know it was bed time. After all, it was 2330. I know I was tired. Lt. Bigger would stay up and watch TV while the rest of us went to bed. Most of us would sleep in our underwear, our bunker pants beside the bed, ready and waiting. I got comfortable under the covers, and then there it was. Dog fart.

There were no runs for Station Four during that night. Station One had two medicals, but we were lucky. I had fallen asleep to dog fart fumes and I awoke to dog breath and a dog tongue in my mouth. Let me tell you, that will wake you up quicker than an alarm clock.

When I got up, the rich aroma of coffee battled the stinky stench of dog. I poured my cup of coffee and sat at the table. It seemed that Bugsy was not the only one with gas.

"All right, who died?" complained Bruce. He always said that when someone stank. "*You* are rotten," Bruce accused me.

"Not me," I answered. We would go back and forth like that.

Lt. Bigger put down his cup and looked at me and asked, "Why don't you go to the neighbor and ask if you could buy Bugsy and just take him home?"

Everyone knew about my special bond with that dog. After a moment, I replied "I should, I guess."

"He runs back and forth between his home and here near busy roads," the lieutenant pointed out.

"I've been thinking about that," I agreed. "I'll go over there today and ask."

Bugsy spent most of the time at the station anyway. He only went home when no one was here. At 0800 I said bye to both units and petted Bugsy before getting in my truck.

As I drove away, I could see Bugsy heading for home, which reminded me to ask his owner if I could buy him. I turned my truck around and drove to the log cabin where his owner lived. I knocked on the door. I heard scratching on the other side, then a bark. When the door opened, Bugsy greeted me by jumping up, his paws on my shoulders and licking my face.

"Looks like you guys know each other," said Mr. Jackson.

"Yes," I said, "I play ball with him at the station."

"Yeah, he stays there a lot," he acknowledged. "What can I do for you?"

"I was wondering if I could buy him from you?" "How much do you want to pay?" he asked. "How about one hundred dollars?"

"No," he snapped, "he's not for sale." He closed the door. That was it. I couldn't buy him, but I knew I'd see him at the station. You can't win 'em all.

# Chapter 14 - Instinct

"Did you see the construction on Commerce Road?" John asked me when I arrived at Station Four for my shift.

"No, I came in the other way," I replied.

"They have Commerce Road shut down," he explained. "They are putting in sewers." Just as he was finishing the last word, the tones went off.

"Station Three and Station Four. You have a possible cave-in at the dig site on Commerce Road. Go to Commerce and Green Lake Road. There will be someone there to show you where to go. Time out, 0855."

"That didn't take long. They just started digging today!" Lt. Bigger commented as we ran to the watch room. John wrote the time and roads down and we hurried to our trucks while the doors rolled up. As the watchman for the day, it was my responsibility to drive the Engine. I started up the big diesel vehicle and pulled the big red truck out. The Rescue was right behind us.

"Engine Four and Rescue Four responding," Lt. Bigger called to dispatch. As he replaced the mic on the dash, the dispatcher responded.

"Message received, Engine Four."

As I was turning right onto Hiller Road, Lt. Bigger turned to me and said, "Engine Three will be there before us." Station Three was at Green Lake and Commerce Roads. Then a voice came over the radio saying "Engine Three responding from Kroger's." So they wouldn't be first on the scene after all.

"It's going to be that kind of day," I said to Lt. Bigger. We turned right on Commerce and saw a man, dressed in yellow reflective clothing, waving his arms to signal us.

"Station One responding," we heard over the radio. On a construction accident involving heavy equipment, Station One customarily responded.

"Engine Four and Rescue Four on scene," Lt. Bigger said as we came to a stop. We were the first responders to arrive. We scrambled out and raced over to a dig site.

The man in yellow waved his arms, yelling, "There is one man down there!" He pointed into a trench. They were supposed to lay sewer pipes, but this hole was way too big for that. The crater was about fifty feet wide and fifteen feet deep. The side closest to us was not steep, but the far side was vertical.

Lt. Bigger's job was to stay atop and run the scene. I grabbed a shovel from the side compartment of the Engine and raced down the side. Rich and Mike were close behind me. On the far ridge of the crater was another worker, pointing down right below him and yelling something to us that we couldn't hear because of the loud growls of the heavy equipment.

Although I couldn't understand him, I knew what he was trying to say. I ran to the spot where he was pointing and saw a fresh pile of dirt. I dropped the shovel and got down on my knees, clawing away the dirt with my hands.

I soon uncovered a man's head. Dirt and mud covered his face and hair. He took a small breath, looking at me with desperation. His bloodshot eyes told me that he could barely breathe. He would not last for long unless something changed quickly.

The guys from the Rescue brought shovels, too. More importantly, they brought oxygen. I turned on the $O_2$ valve and attached the tubing, placing the mask over the man's face while the other two
firefighters kept digging. The man was buried from the neck down, in an upright standing position. All three of us were frantically scooping dirt away, trying to free him.

Engine Three arrived and Lt. Bigger put them on the job of shoring up the sides of the hole. Where we dug, dirt and rocks started to fall around us. I looked up. The side wall was visibly vibrating. Small rocks and sand were sliding into the hole that we were creating. It was an uphill battle to free the worker.

I realized that the vibrations were coming from the heavy equipment that was still running. I looked up at Lt. Bigger and pointed to the diesel equipment, signaling for him to shut it down. He gave me thumbs up to confirm that he understood, and I went back to work.

As we were digging, Engine One and Rescue One arrived. It was a good thing, too, because two workers who came down to try to help their friend ended up hurt themselves. The second we saw them in the hole, we yelled for them to get back up. But before the equipment was moved, a few large chunks of clay and dirt came crashing down the side of the crater and right on top of the two workers. The debris struck one squarely on the head and grazed the other on the shoulder. Both men collapsed in a plume of dust.

At least they had helmets on, or the one man would have had his head taken off. All the same, they were both seriously injured. The heavy equipment was finally rolled back, and the noise stopped. The only clamor now came from the chatter of the radios.

Station Two had just arrived on the scene, so most of the fire department was there. Rescue One's crew worked on the men that had been struck by the chunks of clay, while those of us from Four continued to try freeing the buried worker. Station Two's crew helped Engine Three shore up the loose wall next to us.

There were four of us working to dig out the patient, but we seemed to be getting nowhere. Whatever we dug out caved right back in. Sand is soft and just slides back to the lowest point. Despite our frustration, we *were* making headway. Finally, we got the sand away from the victim's chest so he was able to breathe more freely.

Even so, he was still having a hard time breathing. When I looked up, I noticed a news truck and a camera man filming us. It's a good thing we had helmets on, because bigger rocks were falling on us while the other crew was working to shore up the side with plywood.

Finally, we got the sand off the trapped worker's abdomen, and he felt a lot better. He was still stuck, though, and we had a hard time freeing his lower body. We had to be careful because when we would dig there was danger of jabbing the patient with the shovels and causing further injury.

The Station Two crew had secured the other injured workers to backboards and bandaged their injuries. I noticed that the one guy, who had been hit directly on the head, had a depressed fracture of his skull. He probably had neck injuries, too. The other man had a fractured shoulder and possible neck and back injuries.

They were both put into Stokes baskets and pulled up the side with ropes. The sides of the trench were now secure, and we could work without fear of more cave-ins. We decided to dig a bigger hole around the worker to get his legs out.

Rich had called the hospital and they ordered us to start an IV and give sodium bicarbonate. The hospital doctor said that being buried is like being crushed, and when a person has been crushed for a length of time, no blood is getting in or out of the legs. Then, when the legs are finally released, there is a massive rush of lactic acid in the blood from the extremities to the rest of the body, which can send the patient into cardiac arrest. So, by releasing the man, we could kill him at the same time.

"Well, I hope this works," Rich said, pushing the amp of sodium bicarbonate into the IV. Finally we freed his legs, picked him up out of the hole and placed him on the backboard contained in the stokes basket. We tied the rope to all four corners of the basket and secured the line at the top of the crater. We hoisted the man in the basket up to the top, with the help of the firefighters above.

Once the patient was safely up, we scaled the side of the hole as well. We saw that the patient was just reaching the Rescue vehicle, so we rushed over to help take the patient on the backboard out of the Stokes basket to place him inside the vehicle. Rich and I got in the back and Mike drove.

When we started moving, the force of acceleration pushed us back and to the side. We regained control and examined the patient, as our sirens wailed and the air horns blared. We were pushed around a bit, but that's part of the experience of riding in the back.

Rich was on the radio with the hospital. The doctor ordered us to give another amp of sodium bicarbonate and to also cut off the patient's clothes to examine him top to bottom. We did as we were told.

The patient had scratches all over his body, but he seemed ok. He didn't talk much on the way to the hospital, where we were greeted by the local news crews asking questions.

"He is doing fine. He can't talk right now. I can't answer questions right now. You will have to talk to the doctor," we responded to some of the questions directed at us. We wheeled the worker into the ER, where security stopped the press from following us. Then we delivered the patient to the ER crew.

I told the doctor, "The patient didn't speak, but he was conscious. We gave him two amps of sodium bicarbonate as directed. And his vitals were good."

"Good," replied the doctor, "maybe he will make it. Time will tell." The doctor walked into the trauma room, and we went to the nurses' station to do the paper work. That had been an exhausting run, and we were grateful to catch our breath.

When we returned to Station Four, I noticed the Captain's car parked in front of a closed bay door. When we came to a stop, I got out of the back and the Captain approached me.

"Johnson, I want to talk to you in the bunk room."

"Oh boy," I thought to myself. Aloud I asked, "What did I do this time?"

"We'll talk in the bunk room," was his solemn reply.

My heart sank as I followed him to what we called the "wood shed." When the Captain wanted to talk in the bunk room, we knew that it meant trouble. This time it was me walking in, although for the life of me I had no idea why. I almost felt like a schoolboy about to be scolded by his teacher.

The metal door to the bunk room automatically shut behind us. The room was dark, even with the lights on. As my eyes adjusted to the low light, the Captain spoke.

"Why did you run down in the trench before the sides were secured? You could have been caught in a cave-in and been buried yourself. Then we would have had two or more of you to rescue, because Mike and Rich followed you in."

"Captain, if I hadn't gone down there, that worker would have died."

"Maybe so, but if there had been a cave-in, we would have two or three or more deaths," the Captain pointed out. "And what about the other two workers that followed you in and got injured?"

I was stunned. I thought it had been a good rescue. I replied, "We told the foreman to keep his men out. They went in any way and we yelled at them to get out."

"Well, you're lucky it turned out well," the Captain said.

"I'm glad it turned out well, too," I answered.

"Now, get cleaned up," he ordered as he walked out. The metal door slammed shut behind him, like a final reproach.

Of course all the guys were waiting outside the door, eager to hear what had happened. There were two doors in the bunk room. One went out to the apparatus room where the Captain had exited, and the other led to the kitchen, where the boys and Bugsy were waiting for me.

"Well?" said Lt. Bigger, "what did he want?"

"He said I should not have gone in the trench before it was shored up."

"That's bullshit!" screamed Mike. "It took forty-five minutes before it was shored up. The guy wouldn't have made it."

"And why just you? We went in there too."

"And it could have taken longer if we hadn't had the wood on hand."

Then Lt. Bigger said, "Maybe he has a point. There could have been multiple casualties. Maybe we shouldn't just go diving in to a situation without thinking it through." Then he added, "Still, it was a good save."

It was nice that the guys always had my back. The noon news report came on the TV.

"Look!" announced Rich. "There's the trench!"

The news showed the cave-in site and some of us. The reporter on scene said, "West Bloomfield Fire Department rescued a construction worker who was completely buried. Fire personnel dove right into action, freeing the man and saving his life without thinking of their own safety. Two other workers were also injured, and are in fair condition."

Then the picture flashed to the hospital. "The rescued worker is doing well."

Then the reporter shoved the mic in the patient's face and asked,

"How do you feel?"

He said, "I feel fine. Just embarrassed." "Why are you embarrassed, sir?" she asked.

"Did they have to cut all of my clothes off?" he responded.

So it ended with that. We saved his life and he and the news are focused on how we cut off his clothes. That was all right. We never cared about publicity. We just wanted to do our job and to not be sued.

# Chapter 15 - Family Feuds

I was making a list of groceries for our late lunch and dinner at Station Four when the phone rang. "Station Four, Lt. Bigger speaking." After a pause I heard, "Ok, Chief. I will get him." John pointed to me. By the look in his eyes, I could tell that I might be in trouble. I took the phone and said, "Hi, Chief."

"Hey, Johnson. Do you remember the PIA last year at Maple and Green Road? The 68 year-old man had a stroke in his car and passed out, causing the crash?"

"Ah, yes," I answered, "I think so. He crashed into a tree, right?"

"That's the one," the Chief confirmed. "Well, he died and now the family is suing everyone. You will need to come into Station One and then to Oakland County Circuit Court for a deposition."

"When, Chief?" I asked him.

"When do you work next?" he asked. "Tomorrow."

"Ok, then be here at 0800 hours to get ready for court by 1100." "I'll be there," I promised.

As I hung up the phone, everyone was looking at me.

Lt. Bigger was the first to speak. "What did you do now, Johnson?"

"Wrong run, wrong place, I guess," I answered. "I have to go shopping, but when I get back, I will tell you all about it."

The lieutenant said to me, "You might as well forget about making lunch. It is after 1430 already. Besides, we have some dogs in the fridge."

He noticed the dog sat next to him. "Sorry Bugsy," he said as he petted the dog. The lieutenant added, "And then you can just go out for dinner."

"Ok," I said, nodding, "if that's what everyone wants."
Everyone nodded their approval. "Well let's sit and have a cup of joe and talk."

We sat down at the dinner table, and I told them about the run with the old man as best as I could remember. We have so many runs, it's sometimes hard to remember them all.

"We got a call for a PIA at Maple and Green Roads sometime last year. Engine One and Rescue One responded," I began the story. "I was riding shot gun in the Rescue, so I did the medical report." I took a sip of coffee and continued.

"Anyway the Engine got there first and parked next to a mid- sized car that had crashed into a tree. We parked the Rescue behind the engine. A few cop cars were there, too. Just as we got the equipment out of the Rescue, another car drove up and parked next to us. Out of the car stepped an older woman, which I assumed was the wife. A younger woman and man followed. His kids I think," I added.

"They flew out of the car right to the accident scene before the police were able to get them back. The accident victim was trapped in the car, which had crashed head-on into the tree. Car verses tree and the tree won." I paused here, expecting the others to at least chuckle, but no one did. Except Rich, who always thinks dark humor is funny. I went ahead with the story.

"Anyway, he was trapped in the car and was not breathing. We put in an airway so he could breathe. While we were working on him, the Engine crew got out the Jaws of Life and ripped the door off the car. We short-boarded him, extracted him from the car, then put him on a long board and into the ambulance. He arrested, but we defibrillated him and got him back. Then we took him to the hospital."

"Good save," someone said.

"Oh, yes," said Lt. Bigger, "I remember that run. I was here listening to it on the radio." The lieutenant looked puzzled and asked, "So what was the problem?"

"The problem was," I answered, "that the family members at the scene said that the patient had called them and told them that he was having a stroke. He asked them to help him. So, instead of calling us, they raced to Maple and Green where they found him crashed into a tree. Then they were restrained by the police because they were in the way. We had one Engine, one Rescue, two police cars, an ambulance and their car on the scene."

"So what?" Mike chimed in.

"So," I continued, "they claim that the car crash was caused by the stroke and the brain injury was, in fact, caused by the exhaust from the Engine, the Rescue, the cop cars and the ambulance. In short, every vehicle but theirs was to blame. They are suing GM for manufacturing the Rescue and Engine, they are suing the ambulance company, the police and us." After a pause, I added, "And maybe me."

"They are suing everyone to see what sticks," someone pointed out. I finished the story. "The patient was bedridden until he died. We'll see what happens. I have to admit, I'm a little worried, but I know we did everything by the book."

There was silence as everyone considered what I had told them. I got up from the table and said, "Well, I think I will get lunch started." Then, the tones went off.

"Or not," I said sarcastically.

"Station Four, you have a possible domestic dispute at Roy's Ranch off of Walnut Lake and Haggerty Road. Police are enroute. Time out, 1433."

"Engine Three is still out on a smoke investigation, so all three of you go," Lt. Bigger ordered.

"We've been there before," Rich said. We went to the watch desk where Lt. Bigger gave Rich the paper with the time and address on it. Then we were on our way. I was third man on the Rescue, which meant riding in the back again.

We took Hiller to Green Lake Road to Haggerty to Walnut Lake Road, where there was an old riding stable that had been there for years. In fact, I remember going for a horseback ride there when I was a young kid.

"We've been here a lot lately," Rich commented. Walnut Lake Road coming off of Haggerty was, and still is, a dirt road. When we turned onto Walnut Lake, the truck kicked up stones and dust. I could hear stones bouncing off the bottom on the underside. Out the back window I could see a cloud of dust following close behind us.

We didn't have to go very far before we were there. We pulled up the old dirt driveway with the plume of dust following. The police arrived at the same time. "Rescue Four on scene," announced Rich. We stepped out of the truck and dust enveloped us for a moment. I picked up the trauma kit and $O_2$, handing it off to Mike.

I grabbed the LIFEPAK as the dust cloud dissipated. In front of us was an old, weathered gray farmhouse with no paint left on it. There were two barns behind the house where the horses were kept. At one time it was a great place to go riding, but now it was old and broken down. Even the horses were sad looking.

As we walked up to the wooden screen door, I had to kick a rooster out of the way. It ran away, crowing. I opened the old wooden screen door, causing the ancient spring on it to make a stretching sound. After we all were in, I let go of the door, which sprang shut with a loud bang. The door bounced back open about six inches and then closed with a second, lesser bang.

Standing in front of us was an old woman of about eighty-five. She carried an empty plastic gallon jug in her hand. Under her feet was an eighty-eight year old man, who was unconscious and soaking wet. "He hit me first!" she screamed at us. "So, I let him have it, with this." She held up the plastic jug, its bottom blown out.

I knelt by the elderly man. At least he was breathing. We were checking his vitals when a police officer asked, "Ma'am, can you tell me what happened?"

"Sure I can," she answered. "The bastard threatened to hit me if I didn't shut up, so I took this water jug and smacked him across the face with it." She said proudly, holding up the now empty water jug, its bottom piece swinging free.

Her husband was lying in a puddle of water on the worn wood floor that was covered by a tatty old brown throw rug. The officer said to her, "Ma'am, let's go outside so we can talk."

"Sure, why not?" she agreed in a haughty voice.

The officer walked her to the door. As he opened the door, the older man groaned. She stopped, turned and said to the body, "Try to hit me, and I'll lay you out again, you old bastard." Then she stepped out the door, letting it bang shut behind her. The ambulance brought the stretcher and a long board in. As we were putting the cervical collar on, Rich said, "I sure wouldn't want to mess with her."

"No! Me either," Mike agreed quickly. "Can you imagine, being hit across the face with a full gallon jug?" he continued. "What's a gallon of water weigh?"

"About eight pounds," I answered as we wheeled him out. We lifted him onto the ambulance. Rich said to me, "If I get that way, shoot me." I smiled as I closed the door.

The old man was fine and later that night went back home. We did end up back at Roy's Ranch quite a few more times until the old man died. Then the horses were sold, the property was bought and everything was torn down. Now Walnut Creek Middle School is there. So if I asked any of the newer guys about Roy's Ranch, they would have no idea what I was talking about. Times change, I guess.

When we returned to Station Four, the backup alarm beeped as we eased into our stall. I hopped out of the back and Lt. Bigger met me at the door.

"I just got a call from the Chief. He wants you to call him back."

I went to the phone and dialed the Chief, worried about what he might have to say. He answered the call saying "I have good news! You don't have to go to court tomorrow."

"Good!" I replied, feeling relieved. "Why not?" I asked.

"Because the lawyer of the family advised them not to sue the Fire Department or the Police Department," the Chief explained. "It wouldn't be a winnable case and would bad PR for them."

"That's good," I said, "one less thing to worry about."

Then I asked the Chief, "What about the others that were named in the law suit?"

"They are still are going ahead with them, even with the ambulance company."

"They'll throw everything against the wall and see what sticks," I commented.

"That's right," the Chief agreed, "but we are off the hook."

That night a pizza was delivered to the station. I never made it to the store, but that was ok by the guys. Remember that I wasn't the best cook of the group. After dinner, we cleaned up and vacuumed the carpet. Then I went outside to the brick wall with Bugsy. We played a good long game of "keep away from the big black dog." I lost. I wanted to see how far Bugsy could go, so I threw the ball way over the wall, and over the wall in one bound went Bugsy.

"It might take him a while to find it this time," I thought to myself just as Bugsy leapt back over the wall and dropped the ball at my feet.

Bugsy and I spent the rest of the evening playing our game. After he got tired, he walked over to the slop sink and sat down waiting for me to wet him down with the hose. I finally went back inside and sat down to watch the evening news. I was feeling sleepy.

"I might just go to bed early," I said as I leaned back in the recliner to ponder going to the bunk room. A loud noise was coming from my left. I looked over to the couch where Mike was sitting, asleep with his head back and snoring so loudly that we couldn't hear the TV. Bugsy was sitting at my side looking at Mike.

I said to Bugsy, "Go wake him up!" I pointed at Mike as I said it and Bugsy got the message. The dog jumped from where he was sitting over by my recliner right onto the couch where Mike was sleeping. Mike bounced up into the air when the big black dog hit the couch. Bugsy lay on Mike's lap, licking his slobbery drool all over Mike's face. Didn't I say he was a smart dog?

Mike woke immediately and just lay there, taking the tongue as everyone was laughing. "Mike," I said, "wake up and go to sleep."

Sleep was not in the cards, however. The tones went off.

"Station Four, you have another domestic assault at 1430 River Drive. Time out, 2138. Be advised, I have a patrol car on the way."

We made our way to the watch desk where Lt. Bigger handed Rich the sheet of paper with the address and times, along with the section map. We found the street on the wall map, then rushed to the Rescue. The doors opened as we pulled out.

"Rescue Four enroute."

"Enroute received, Rescue Four."

I was in back, but there was an opening into the front to allow movement if necessary. I could stick my head up front to see what was going on. It was now dark out and the flashing red lights reflected off of the signs along the side of the road.

We made a quick turn to avoid something in the road. The sudden movement threw me into the cabinets on the side of the Rescue. That's why I was supposed to be strapped in the seat. I sat down, buckled my belt and rubbed the new bruise forming on my shoulder.

"Rescue Four on scene." Out the side window, I could see a young man standing beside the road, holding a bloody sheet on his left arm. A woman stood next to him. I opened the side door as we stopped and hopped out.

Mike and Rich were with me as the man and woman approached us. "I cut my arm real f'ing bad," the young man said, pointing at his covered arm.

"Ok," Rich responded. "It's dark out here, so let's get in the Rescue where there is more light."

I got in the back to help the man up. He reached his good arm toward me and I helped pull him in as Mike was steadying him from behind. Once in the truck, the guy sat down on the stretcher. Rich, Mike and the woman climbed in behind him.

"What's your name?" I asked.

"Jack," the man responded, then added, "Look what I did to my f'ing arm!"

I gently unwrapped the bloody sheet from his arm, exposing the injury. To my surprise his bicep muscle was cut in half, right across the middle and down to the bone. His muscle tissue was exposed and on the inside I saw what looked like rings. Basically it looked like what you would see in a steak. I also saw blood vessels, tendons and clotted blood.

The two halves of the biceps pulled apart and started squirting blood all over. Rich had a large trauma dressing ready, which he slapped on the wound as we both held the muscle tightly together. We put a pressure bandage on the wound as well. I told Mike to drive and cancel the ambulance. It would be faster and better for the patient. We got the bleeding under control fairly quickly.

It was clear he would need surgery to put the muscle back together. After we finished bandaging his arm I asked, "How did you injure it?"

"I was pissed off at her for locking me out of the house," he answered. "When she wouldn't open the door, I got so angry I punched through the window with my fist. My arm went most of the way through, and when I was pulling it out I felt the glass slice me. I saw it being cut in half. Blood was everywhere. My girlfriend got me that sheet," he continued.

"I guess I had a bit too much to drink," he admitted. With the smell on his breath, I would say he did, indeed, have too much to drink. I noticed that his girlfriend hadn't said a word.

"She locked me out of my own damn house," he said, looking at her. Finally the woman started talking, and didn't shut up until we arrived at the hospital. The accusations flew back and forth. We tried to calm things down, but they incessantly continued the verbal boxing. Mercifully for all of us, it wasn't long before we arrived at the hospital. The police were waiting for us.

We wheeled the patient into the ER. His girlfriend yapped at him and he swore at her the whole way. I was so glad when we were able hand them over to the nurse and the police.

"I can see why they wanted to kill each other," Rich joked as we were walking to the nurses' station. "Isn't love wonderful?" he added.

"Well," I said, "I think they were made for each other."

"That's why I will never get married," Mike remarked.

"Mike, you *are* married," Rich reminded him.

"Oh yeah, I almost forgot."

As Rich did the medical report, Mike and I went out to the Rescue to clean the blood off the floor and wherever else it had splattered. We scrubbed the truck and put the equipment back in order. It's amazing how a rig gets so messed up on such a short run.

It was interesting that the two domestics we dealt with ran to the extremes. An older, married couple and a young couple, both doing their best to hurt one another verbally and physically. Thank goodness not everyone experiences that kind of love.

# Chapter 16 - Close Encounters

Since I was assigned watch duty, I had to sleep in the watch room. I was responsible for logging all runs, taking all phone calls and making sure everyone was up if a run came in. I also had to get the address and the time of the run recorded, in addition to finding the location on the map.

The worst thing for me was being rattled out of bed for a fire in the early morning hours when it was almost time to go home. So, of course, it happened that night while I was on watch. With the tones shaking us out of our beds, and the bright lights crashing on, I was trying to remember where I was as I came out of a sound sleep. I heard the dispatcher over the radio.

"Station Four, Station Three, Station One, you have a possible structure fire at 5738 Hiller. Time out, 0644."

I was at Station Four, so I and everyone else on duty stumbled into bunker gear. I had already written the address and time on a slip of paper, and was trying to find the cross streets on the map. My eyes were not focusing well yet, but I found the street in section four. Now I had to get out the section map from the map box and find the exact address. That's when everyone got to the watch room.

I handed the information to Lt. Bigger as we headed out the door, pushing the automatic opener before climbing into the vehicle. I drove the Engine out of the stall.

"That's where Bugsy lives!" Lt. Bigger exclaimed, looking at the map. I looked at him, suddenly wide awake, and pulled first onto Greer then left onto Hiller. My heart was racing as we got closer to the house. In my mind I was going over the steps of what to do when we got there.

I was a little nervous because we had just gotten a new Engine. At least we didn't have to worry about Bugsy, because he was already safe at the station.

Lt. Bigger said, "There is a hydrant right in front of the house."

"Ok, Lieutenant. I just hope it works," I said back. That particular hydrant was part of the Zox subdivision water. The water for that sub came from a pumping station it owned. It was very old and unreliable at best. Some of the water pipes were even made of wood! That's how ancient the system was.

It was a very short ride to the house. As I pulled up in front of it, I could see smoke rising from the large barn behind the house. I stopped beside the hydrant, put the pumper into park then pushed the lever for the air brakes. They hissed as they did their job.

Lieutenant Bigger launched out the door. Since it was our run, he would be in charge of the fire. I put the Engine in pump and pulled the PTO to engage the pump. Then I got out and went to the side where Mike and Rich were pulling off the cross-lays. I would help pull off hose if necessary. They had that in hand, so I went to the control panel on the side of the engine.

Over the radio I heard Lt. Bigger say, "We have a working fire in the barn." We had already planned for this scenario, because we knew the barn was used for making hockey sticks. I'm not sure for whom Mr. Jackson was making them, but it was well known that there were plenty of flammable liquids, resins and lots of wood in there.

At the control panel I pulled out the tank-to-pump lever to get the pump started. Then I looked at the hose to make sure that it was straight. Engine Three pulled up and the crew of two helped Mike and Rich stretch out the hose. I had to wait until it was straitened before I turned on the water flow. Otherwise it would kink and stop the water. Once the weight of the water was in the hose, it would be very hard or impossible to unkink.

Once it was all set, I pulled out the pump-to-hose lever. The two and a half and one and a half filled up in a hurry, starting close to the truck and traveling down the hose to the nozzle.

I looked at the pressure gauge on the panel and saw there was about 50 psi on the pump, which was about right. The pumper has a lever and a psi gauge for every hose that the truck can run, which is eight in total.

I had never needed that many, though. Each inch and a half hose is 80 psi at the nozzle. I adjusted the lever to about 90 psi, accounting for friction loss. Any more pressure than that would make it very difficult to control.

The nozzle that we used was a variable stream type. That meant it could be adjusted by twisting to get anything from fog spray for close fires with not much pressure, to a straight stream for spraying water over a long distance with more pressure and power. Even when the nozzle was shut off, it leaked to allow the air out when the hose was filled. It also kept the water moving, so it wouldn't freeze during the winter.

I set the pressures and engaged the governor. The governor makes sure that the pressure stays the same, regardless if someone shuts off or turns on a hose.

Otherwise, there would be a sudden increase or decrease of pressure. A sudden increase of pressure, which we called a "water hammer," could injure someone by knocking him down or even causing a firefighter to lose control of the hose. A decrease of pressure while in a fire could cost a life.

After the hose pressures were set, I went to the front of the pumper and had to hook the front suction to the hydrant. The engine only holds five hundred gallons of water. In a big fire you may run out of water fast, so we connect to a hydrant. That was the idea anyway, but as I said, this hydrant wasn't always reliable.

I pulled the big yellow five-inch suction hose off the front bumper and hauled it to the hydrant. Using the hydrant wrench, I twisted off the cap and connected the suction hose to it. Then, making sure there were no kinks in the suction hose, I secured the hydrant wrench to the lug on top of the hydrant. I twisted it open.

To my relief, the suction hose filled. Then I went back to the panel and pushed closed the tank-to-pump lever while pulling open the suction-to-pump lever at the same time. Sometimes the pressure from the hydrant is more or less than what the pump pressure is, so after opening the hydrant the pressure has to be adjusted again.

Everything was now ready! I had to continuously monitor the gauges and then grease the pump bearings. I figured that at some time in the near future, we would need to add a two and one half line. In addition to all of this, I had to keep track of what equipment was taken off the truck.

"Rescue Four is entering the building," called Lt. Bigger. There was a big door that had to be breeched before they could enter the barn. I watched from the Engine while the firefighters entered the building. I guess the barn was insulated since it was used in the winter. That at least explained what happened next.

The door of the barn was not locked, and it opened easily. Smoke poured out the door as two firefighters in full gear and SCBA entered the barn with an inch and one half hose and disappeared into the darkness. They were in for about ten seconds when the smoke outside the barn started to be drawn back in.

It was just a little at first, but then smoke was sucked into the barn faster and faster. A big rush of air swept in through the barn door, pulling in paper, leaves and whatever else was close. Everyone watching knew what was happening. "Get out! Get out of the barn now!" people began yelling.

It was too late. Booooom! A huge explosion tore through the air. Fire shot out of the barn like a cannon blast. Wood, smoke, embers and two firefighters were ejected from the barn. The firefighters tumbled head over heels, rolling right to my feet next to the Engine. Both of their masks and helmets had been ripped off.

I was stunned. I never saw anything like that before. One of the worst situations a firefighter can get into is a backdraft or flashover. I had just witnessed a terrifying event that has historically caused the deaths of many firefighters. I looked in disbelief at my colleagues lying on the ground.

As I knelt down to check them out, one suddenly shouted, "What the hell happened?" It was Mike.

"I think we are still alive," said the other one, who turned out to be Rich. Unbelievably, they seemed ok as they picked themselves up from the ground. Lt. Bigger came running up, terror in his eyes.

"Are you ok?" he asked incredulously.

"I guess so, Chief," Rich said, blowing smoke out of his mouth. Rescue One's crew was running our way. They were relieved when they saw that the guys appeared to be all right. The lieutenant ordered Mike and Rich into Rescue One to be evaluated.

After they left for the hospital, the lieutenant looked at me and said, "I thought they were dead." I must admit, so had I, but they were fine. Thank the Lord! Everything turned out ok that time.

The thing about explosions is they can extinguish the fire that caused them, and that is exactly what happened in this case. It's like blowing out a match.

The barn fire was out, but it still had to be overhauled and all the hot spots cooled off. My father-in-law was there on scene, since he was a volunteer firefighter. He came up to me at the Engine and said, "Greg, there is an airplane in the barn. I hit my head on the wing. You should go in and take a look."

I did go in later and sure enough it was an airplane wing. The barn was full of all sorts of junk besides an aircraft and hundreds of hockey sticks. There were bundles of wood to make the sticks, all sorts of cans of glue and fiberglass resin, and things like propane tanks and cans of paint. I could go on and on. One big fire hazard.

We spent the rest of the time putting out hot spots. I was on overtime now because it was after 0800. Unit Two took over engineering the pumper. Lt. Bigger said to me, "Let's get in the utility truck and return to the station."

When we pulled in, John said to me, "Don't forget to fill out the overtime sheet." He pulled out two forms from the drawer and handed one to me. We filled them out and put them into the basket designated for Station One.

I turned to John and asked, "What is the last you heard about Mike and Rich?"

"I heard they are doing fine," John answered. "They have some minor burns, cuts and bruises, but they should be going home today."

"That's great!" I was relieved. That was the closest anyone came to being killed in the Department while I worked there.

I was glad to finally have an extended bit of time off. I had traded Kelly days with someone, which meant I would have to pay it back in November, but for now, it was worth it. I was heading up north. I had kissed my wife and my little boys goodbye.

"So, you want to go up norff with me?" I had asked my wife. Up norff was our family nickname for the place.

"No way. That place stinks." She did have a point. The house trailer we owned did smell musty. It had been made in 1954, so it was already old when I got it. I owned ten acres up in Salba, Michigan. When I was a kid, my parents bought the property and moved the trailer there. Later, my father sold it to me.

So, there I was, without wife or kids, going up norff to get it ready for hunting season. I liked to go up there in late July to cut the grass, clean up and plant corn to attract deer. It was a four hour trip, but I didn't mind the drive.

The only things in Salba itself were a bar, a party store and a gas station. And the gas station went out of business, if that tells you anything. I should mention there's a fire department as well.

As I reached the Salba town limits there, in the middle of the only major intersection where M-32 crosses Gaylord Road, I encountered a cattle hauler semi on its side. The wheels were still spinning.

I pulled my truck over to the shoulder of the road and approached the overturned semi. The cattle trailer was closest to me, and I saw a cow pulling itself out of the wreckage, mooing as she escaped. Then another cow pulled herself out as I walked by. I looked between the slats and saw cows lying dead and mangled inside. I couldn't worry about the cows escaping with a man still in the cab, so I let them go.

Just as I got to the cab, the Salba Fire Department arrived. The Chief came up to me as I was checking on the unconscious driver.

"What are you doing?" he demanded. I could tell he was Chief because he was wearing a white helmet.

"I'm a firefighter paramedic from West Bloomfield Fire Department," I told him.

"We don't have any paramedics here. We've got this," he said by way of dismissal.

Other volunteers had started to arrive in their small pickups with the big light bars.

"If you want to help, direct traffic in the intersection," the Chief ordered. I wondered whether I should do it or not. It *was* their run…Oh, what the heck. I walked over to the intersection and prepared to direct traffic. I waited quite a while before a car finally came through. I duly pointed which way to go.

From behind me a female called out, "Hey! That's my job!" I turned around and saw a woman who couldn't have been more than five foot tall, her one leg shorter than the other. She held a stop sign in her hand. She limped up to me and repeated, "This is my job!"

I could not believe this! "Ok," I replied, trying not to offend her further, "go ahead. Take it!" I walked back in frustration towards the cattle hauler. A lot of cows had escaped and were now disappearing into the woods.

I wandered up to the cab again, where two Salba firefighters were talking to the injured driver. "You sure you don't need any help?" I asked again.

"We don't have paramedics here!" the Chief, snapped, clearly irritated at my presence. Just then a paramedic unit ambulance arrived from Mancelona, which was about twenty miles away. As the Mancelona paramedics got out of their truck, I climbed into mine.

I drove past the woman holding the sign, past the escaping cows and towards my property. Sometimes reality is simply stranger than fiction.

I pulled onto the grass-covered driveway. My ten acres were in the middle of nowhere. All around my trailer were mostly woods and some meadow. Across the dirt road was an eighty-acre field that had been bought and sold many times over the years.

The last time anyone had lived there was the previous year. A guy had brought in a broken down house trailer and tried to fix it while he was living there. He had left all sorts of trash scattered around the eighty acres; refrigerators, propane tanks, old cars and a lot of garbage. I stood looking at the mess briefly then went back to my side of the road. I did what I came up there for.

About two hundred yards into the woods behind my trailer is where I hunted. I cut the grass, tilled the ground and planted it with corn. I looked down. At my feet I saw enormous deer tracks. The ground was sandy, so it was easy to follow them to the edge of the woods. There, just inside the tree line, were the largest deer I'd ever seen. I crept closer. I could hear a dull metallic ding sound.

As I got nearer, I could see that it might not be a deer. The huge beast started walking towards me, and the dull ding sound grew louder. I couldn't help thinking that it sounded like a cow bell. Then the beast came into focus. Yes, it was indeed a cow bell, attached to one of the escaped cows.

I wondered if I should catch it and lead it back to town. I moved towards it, but the cow must have seen what I was going to do. She turned around and ran back into the woods, mooing and clanging the cow bell as she disappeared. The cow had made a lucky escape. I wasn't about to chase her.

"Shows to go ya what happens when you try to help," I said aloud to myself, using my trademark mixed-up version of the popular saying.

The sun was starting to get low in the sky. I decided to sit in my tree stand, some twenty feet off the ground, and watch to see if the deer would come in to nibble the corn. I enjoyed just being outside and observing the wildlife.

At dusk, I was rewarded with the sight of six deer wandering out. I watched them as they walked by, always looking around and sweeping their tails. They would put their heads down to get a bite of grass and corn, then jerk their heads up to listen and look. They would wag their tails and then bend their heads back down to eat some more.

As the deer wandered away, it started to drizzle. I hadn't expected it to rain, but that's Michigan weather for you. Things were starting to get wet, and I knew it was time to get down. I began my descent, placing my foot on a knot on the tree the way I always did.

My hands slipped from the wet tree stand at the same time my foot slipped. I grasped the thick branch just in reach below me. I wrapped my arms around it and felt it snap under my weight. I plunged head first down the tree. Everything happened in slow motion. I wasn't worried because I always thought I would be able to catch myself.

I clutched at another thick branch and was able to arrest my fall. But it, too, snapped off, sending me into free fall again. There were no more branches to grab, so I snatched at the trunk of the tree to try to ride it down. Small branches snapped off as I fell.

All of a sudden, I stopped; my head dangled about one foot off the ground. What had stopped me? It was a metal tree step that I had fastened into the tree trunk to help me climb up to the stand. I was suspended upside down, my arms wrapped around the tree trunk and my clothes hung up on the metal step.

I eased myself down and sat on the ground for a minute to catch my breath and collect my thoughts. When I felt a little steadier, I got to my feet and brushed myself off. I was thinking, "I guess I got away with it that time."

I didn't hurt anywhere, but as I was brushing the dirt off my sweatshirt, I noticed a large tear in the sleeve. I opened the rent in the fabric and looked inside.

"Oh boy!" I said aloud, seeing blood flowing out of a large v-shaped gash in my forearm. I took off my sweatshirt to examine the wound. I wiped the blood off with the fabric, and I could see the muscle in my forearm. It didn't seem to be bleeding much, but as I looked closer I could see blood vessels and tendons. It was like the injury the guy who put his arm through the glass door ended up with.

I wrapped the sweatshirt around my arm and started back to my trailer. It was an uphill walk, which I had never noticed until now. I wanted to take it easy because I didn't know for sure how bad I was bleeding. It took me ten minutes to get back to the trailer. I grabbed my car keys and drove myself towards the hospital.

Then I realized I had no idea where the hospital was. I saw the Salba party store to my right and decided to stop and get directions. I entered the store, which looked like a well-preserved turn of the century establishment, my shoes clopping on the wooden floor. The bells chimed, alerting the cashier to my presence.

She was in her forties, and was ringing up a customer when she noticed me. She slammed the drawer shut as she asked, "May I help you?"

I saw out of the corner of my eye a younger man standing beside the main door, leaning against a wall. "Can you tell me how to get to a hospital?" I asked.

"The closest one is in Gaylord, about thirty miles away." She looked at my arm wrapped in a bloody sweatshirt. Then she asked me the dreaded question.

"Do you want me to call the fire department?"

I thought back to the way they had treated me earlier that day as I answered, "No, thank you. I've seen them in action."

The man at the door spoke, slurring his words, "I can I-I can dr-drive you if-if-if you want." He was obviously drunk.

"No, thanks, I can drive myself. Besides, I need my truck." I tried to sound grateful for the offer so as not to offend.

So the lady gave me directions to the hospital, and I was on my way. In the emergency room I was met by a nurse who led me to a treatment area. The ER doctor was a woman, and she cleaned up my wound by sticking her gloved hand in my open flesh under the skin flap to make sure there was no dirt left inside. That was the most painful part. Next a neurosurgeon came in to see what neurological damage I may have sustained.

He told me, "You should be proud of yourself! You are the first patient I have had that fell out of a tree stand that did not receive a spinal injury."

I was shocked! The nurse injected me in the armpit to numb my arm. The neurosurgeon said I would stay awake while he sewed up my arm, but I didn't. I guess all of the stress, in addition to the physical work I'd done that day, had caught up with me.

When I awoke, I was in a hospital room. My wife had been called and told what had happened. The neurosurgeon came in to see me and told me I had been given sixty stitches. He then told me I could go home tomorrow but could not go back to work for a month. He wished me luck as he walked out. My right arm was in a splint and heavily bandaged.

"I guess I won't be working for a while." I thought. About 3:00 am, I was awakened by a sharp pain in my left leg. We had all been so concerned with my arm that we had forgotten the rest of me. I could feel a large baseball-sized knot in my left leg by my groin. I was just now starting to feel pains all over my body.

I was thinking, "Man, I could still be lying under that tree and no one would know where I was." What the surgeon had said about having spinal injuries worried me in particular. I prayed a lot that night, thanking the Lord for sparing my life and preventing worse injuries.

After I was checked out, I looked at the knot in my leg. It was a large hematoma. Blood was seeping under my skin and down my leg. When I was released, I got in my truck and drove home one-handed.

The long ride gave me time to think about the fall. How it happened in slow motion, and how I never felt I was in any real trouble. And when I found out I was ok, I thought I had done a good job saving myself. The reality that the accident could have left me lying under the tree, with no one the wiser, was very unsettling. After all, no one expected me home for three days.

By the time I got home, my leg was in great pain. This time when I checked my bruise, I could see that the black and blue had run from my upper thigh down to my ankle. It looked cool!

I was off work for a month. When I got the splint and bandages off, the stitches had left a large v-shaped scar on my forearm, just under my elbow. You've heard the old saying "Chicks dig scars?" Not true!

# Chapter 17 - Friction

I was sometimes scheduled at Station Nine. This station did not originally belong to West Bloomfield, but had been part of the Tri-City Volunteer Department. It consisted of three cities: Sylvan Lake, Orchard Lake and Keego Harbor. It had been volunteer-based since before I was born. Eventually, the citizens of Tri-City wanted a full-time fire and paramedic department. It took many years to achieve, with the volunteers fighting to maintain their status quo. When it finally happened, it was sudden.

Almost overnight, West Bloomfield had three more cities to cover. The volunteers were not happy, and I can't blame them. The change gave us a new station, pumper and Rescue.

One Sunday when I was there, it turned out to be a lazy day, with nothing much happening. I was in charge of the station, and we had a new rookie. I conducted a drill and took the rookie out twice to drive the pumper for practice and to learn the streets. The other fellas weren't too happy with me, but I also put on a station drill.

I learned that we would start hose testing the next day. I was grateful to know I was scheduled off. Hose testing was tedious work, but since it usually lasted a week or more, I knew I wasn't off the hook completely.

On Tuesday, I was on watch. I was supposed to go shopping, make the meals and then help with hose testing at Station Four. So, that's what I did. The process involved getting out all of the rolled-up hose. Each roll was fifty feet long. We unrolled them outside and hooked them together, then connected them to the Engine.

Next, we pressurized the hose for about five minutes. Finally, we shut off the pump, drained the water, uncoupled all the hose, rolled it up, and carried it back to the apparatus room. Each hose had to be cleaned in a hose washer and dryer before we put it away and recorded whether it had passed or failed.

In addition to this, we had to take the two thousand feet of two and a half inch hose off the back of the Engines, plus all the other hose that was stored there, test it and reload it all. It could take up to two weeks to complete. We would usually get together with another station to accomplish this big task.

On the day I was on watch, Station Four and Station Three worked to get Engine Three's hoses changed. With Station Three there, I would have to go if we had a medical, even though I was on watch and assigned to the Engine. It was not a bad thing when the medical calls came in. I wasn't unhappy when I had to leave that work.

"Stations Two and Four, you have a boating accident at the boat launch on Pleasant Lake. A Sea-Doo has hit a dock. Time out, 1055 hours. Please be advised police are enroute."

Lt. Bigger yelled, "I want Three to go!" So I pulled my gear off the Engine and hopped into the back of the Rescue. The apparatus room doors were already open as we went out. We all knew where the boat launch was, so we didn't need a map.

"Rescue Four enroute with Three," said Rich.

"Enroute with Three received, Rescue Four."

"Engine Two responding."

"Engine Two responding received," echoed dispatch.

Engine Two arrived at the boat launch just before we did. They were getting out of the rig as we parked the man met us when we got out of the truck. I could see in his face that there was a bad situation ahead.

He led us to the lake behind a multimillion dollar house that sat next to the boat launch. "We were riding Sea-Doos," the guy said. "I saw the dock and I went around it, but my buddy didn't." Although no one had asked him, he answered, "And yes, he had been drinking, but I haven't."

He led us down to a long metal dock that stretched out into the lake. The sun reflected off the water into our eyes, which made things difficult to see until we crouched under the dock and out of the bright light. I could smell the fishy water scent carried in by the slight breeze. I have always liked that smell, associating it with good times. Not that day, though.

Lying under the dock was a twenty-two year old man, a kid really, who was in great pain. His Sea-Doo was drifting away on the other side of the dock, disappearing into the reflected sunshine.

The guy was trying not to yell out in pain, he just grimaced until it became too much. His back was on the sandy shore, and his legs were in about a foot of water. His legs looked deformed by the accident. He had obviously fractured both femurs, but at least no bone poked through the skin yet.

As we checked him over, we got the story. They had been riding the Sea-Doos one behind the other. The first one saw the dock and turned quickly to avoid it. His buddy saw it too late. His Sea-Doo went under the dock, but both his legs hit it, and so did his head. He was very lucky he wasn't killed instantly.

We have to be careful on these types of injuries, because he had obvious femur fractures to take care of. He could also have had a spinal injury or a head injury, and we would have to treat him for that too.

"My legs! They hurt!" he finally cried out.

"You've broken your legs," Rich told him. "We'll take care of you and get you to the hospital."

"It hurts so bad!"

"I know," Rich soothed him. "We'll get you something for the pain." In general, we don't give pain meds to a patient if there's a chance for a head injury. It can make it harder to determine what's going on. However, when we have to splint a patient's broken legs, we administer pain meds to prevent the person moving them involuntarily due to the pain. That could cause the bones to pop through the skin, creating an even worse injury.

We checked his vitals, and they were good. His blood pressure was a little high, but with the pain he was in, it was to be expected. I gave him a shot of morphine after we started an IV. I never administered meds unless I had an IV in place. With the morphine on board, it didn't take long for the patient to relax.

The Engine crew put a cervical collar on his neck while we worked on his legs. We got two long femur traction splints. We took the patient's foot and pulled to get traction on his leg. He jumped, even with the morphine, because the two sharp ends of the femur bones were rubbing against each other and the tissue inside his
leg. Broken bones are usually sharp and can cut through the skin if they're not handled carefully.

Once the leg was in proper traction, the patient relaxed because the bones were aligned, and the pain was less. We put the traction splint next to his groin. On the other end I attached the cravat on the splint to his foot. We secured the splint to his leg with Velcro straps and then starched it to make it stiff and more supportive.

The traction splint has tubes inside of tubes, which allows you to make the splint longer. It also has notches so it can lock in place. Someone has to keep traction on the leg while the splint is put in place. When the splint is stretched, it locks and then you can let go of the foot.

We did the same to his right leg. We discovered the boy's name was William. Once both splints were in place, he had a big smile on his face. That morphine was great stuff. When the ambulance arrived, they brought over a long back board. All seven of us lifted William onto it and then put him on the stretcher.

As we were pushing the stretcher around the house to the ambulance, I looked over to the police car. William's buddy was bent over the cop car, his hands cuffed behind his back. Then the cop guided him into the back of the patrol car. I guess he had been drinking after all.

During the month I had been off healing from my tree stand injury, there had been some fireworks happening at the department. A new lieutenant had admitted to cheating on his officer's test. He had been given some of the answers ahead of time by another officer. Because of their religious convictions, both men decided to come
in and confess to the Chief about what they had done. They knew it could get them fired.

Needless to say, the Chief was devastated. He didn't fire them, but he gave them a month's suspension with no pay. They both were friends of mine, so I was glad I would be able to see them again.

However, not everyone felt that way. Some people in the department thought they should be fired. Others thought they should have kept their mouths shut and deal with the guilt as punishment in order to spare the fire department the embarrassment.

So ex-lieutenant Jim, who had been in charge at Station One, was now transferred to Station Three because no one wanted to work with him. When Jim arrived, everyone sitting at the table got up and walked out except for me. I guess I stayed put because I kind of knew what he was going through. Being a Christian myself, I could understand wanting to set your mistakes right. And I understood the need to forgive.

Jim came to the table with a cup of coffee, but he just stood there, looking uncomfortable. He finally spoke. "You probably can't stand to look at me," he said meekly.

"Jim," I replied, "it would be an honor to work with you."

"Really?" he asked. I could tell he hadn't been expecting that.

"I understand what happened and I don't care," I explained. "Besides, we have always worked well together." After that we got along fine. It's nice to know someone has your back. Still it was a bit awkward because he had been my boss and now I was his boss.

Jim and I spent all morning at Station Four testing hose. At about 1300, we returned to Station Three. At about 1700, Jim went back to Station Four to help them put away their hose while I put ours away.

Jim returned to Station Three at about 1900, followed soon after by Captain Slasher. The name fit him. He was the type of person that thinks so much of himself that he believes everyone likes and respects him when really they don't.

"Johnson, I want to see you in the apparatus room right now!" Captain Slasher yelled my way.

"Now what?" I wondered. I followed the Captain to the apparatus room, with Jim trailing behind us.

"Why didn't you help with the hose testing today?" the Captain yelled.

"But I did!" I answered, surprised and a little bit irritated at the accusation.

"They told me you didn't help."

Jim jumped in, adding, "He was there helping."

"But you weren't there tonight," Slasher snapped again.

"I was here putting hose away," I explained.

"They told me at Station Four that you didn't want to help," the Captain challenged. Jim jumped to my defense again.

"I volunteered to go over there myself to help while Greg stayed here putting away hose."

"And," Captain Slasher continued as though he hadn't heard Jim, "last Sunday you did nothing at Station Nine. You had a subby, but the guys told me that he didn't have any training."

"That's not true!" I countered. "I took the subby out two times in the Engine, and I gave the whole station a drill, even though it was Sunday."

"That's not what they told me," Slasher said.

Jim chimed in, "Johnson told me that he thought he had a good day at Station Nine. He mentioned that he had trained the boys."

The Captain had had enough. He threatened, "Jim, if you value your job, you will shut up. Go back in the bunk room." Captain Slasher waited until the door slammed behind Jim as he left.

Then he asked, "Why don't you defend yourself?"

I shrugged and answered, "I don't think it matters what I say on this witch hunt. It's clear to me that you have some sort of agenda in mind here. None of these accusations has any merit, but that doesn't really matter, does it?"

Then Slasher asked me, "Why don't you get mad?" I didn't bother to answer. Instead, I just held his gaze.

"You are transferred to Station Two effective tomorrow." Then Slasher turned around, got in his car and left.

A few moments later, Jim walked into the apparatus room to check on me. I told him I was being transferred to Station Two because Slasher knew it was my least favorite. Jim looked concerned for me. "Don't worry, Jim. I'll be fine," I assured him.

Jim called Station Nine and they said they never said those things. Neither did Station Four. So Slasher was lying. Of course, I had already suspected that. In fact, most people that met him thought that he was pure evil. It is said that whatever comes around goes around.

Well Captain Slasher believed he would one day be Assistant Chief and then Chief of the Department. Instead, he ended up being passed over and left the fire department a bitter man.

Sometimes justice *does* prevail.

# Chapter 18 - Dogs

As I mentioned, I didn't care for Station Two much because I didn't know the area as well as the others. In addition, there were a large number of condominiums, so the population density was greater, leading to more runs. Lastly, it seemed that the Rescue was always out on call to one of the many rest homes in Station Two's area. There were lots of little things that were not ideal about that station.

I was met in the parking lot by Lt. Dale, the station officer. He welcomed me by saying, "I heard what was done to you. That sucks, but now you're here."

"Now I am here," I agreed. "Well, Lieutenant, let's go inside and get some coffee."

At Station Two there was only one station officer who worked with me half the time, leaving me in charge the other half. At those times, I would receive "in-charge pay." That kind of pay rate could add up quickly, and I soon figured out that I might make a little extra money working there.

Lt. Dale led the way to the kitchen. I poured myself a cup of joe and sat with the guys and the woman. Kathy was one of a handful of women who worked in our department. I'd been on runs with her before and knew she was a good fire fighter. I could trust her to have my back.

So that made four of us: The lieutenant, Kathy, Me and Bill. It was always a bit awkward for a while when you started at a new station. You don't know the people very well, which could make it hard. With this group, however, I knew I'd be just fine.

"Bill said he would take today's watch," Lt. Dale told me.

"Thanks, Bill," I answered appreciatively.

"You'll be driving the Rescue," Lt. Dale added.

"Sounds good to me," I agreed. The first tones of the shift perked our ears.

"Engine Three, Rescue Two, you have a boating accident at 6534 Long Lake Court, at the public beach. Time out, 0830."

"I haven't even checked out the Rescue yet," I thought to myself. Usually I would have inspected it by now, but with my getting-to-know-you time that morning, no one had checked out their trucks.

"I hope Unit Two put the equipment back today," I said as we ran for the Rescue. The apparatus room door opened and out we went with lights and sirens blaring. Even though we knew approximately where the beach was, Kathy looked it up on the map to make sure.

I picked up the microphone and called in, "Rescue Two responding."

"Engine Three responding," said a voice over the radio. That was the person who had taken my place at that station. Oh well.

"Responding received, Engine Three and Rescue Two," replied the dispatcher.

"Hey, isn't that the same place where your Sea-Doo accident was?" Kathy asked as she put down the map.

"Almost," I answered. "It's the next lot to the south." It was going to be a fairly long ride to the public beach for us, so Station Three arrived before us.

"Engine Three on the scene."

"On the scene received, Engine Three," the dispatcher confirmed. A minute later Engine Three came on the air.

"Rescue Two, we have a severely injured woman on the beach." Kathy picked up the mic and answered, "Ok, Engine Three, we're about one minute out."

When we arrived, I pulled in front of the beach. A chain link fence with a narrow gate provided the only access to the waterfront.

"Rescue Two on scene," Kathy called on the radio. I parked the Rescue and we all stepped out. We quickly grabbed the equipment and squeezed through the narrow gate. A hill, covered in crab-grass and a number of tall oak trees, blocked our view of the accident until we reached the peak. Then we could see the Engine Three crew crouched over someone lying in the water.

We made our way past families having picnics, and a mid-sized speed boat that had been pulled up onto the sandy shore. A man in his thirties and a woman in her late twenties were with the Engine crew. They were all kneeling in the water next to an injured woman.

The fishy water smell grew stronger as we approached. I stepped along on the sand, rushing toward the patient. I knelt with the others in the sandy water.

"What is your name?" I asked the patient.

"Mary," she answered calmly, although she was bleeding. Her right leg had rows of large deep u-shaped lacerations from her upper thigh down to her ankle.

The Engine Three crew was compressing the lacerations that were bleeding the most. "Can you tell us what happened?" Kathy asked, as we got a lot of dressings and gauze out of the trauma box.

"I was driving the boat," the man in the bathing trunks explained, "pulling her skiing and she fell. I turned the boat around to pick her up, but I guess I got too close and hit her with the prop."

The rows of gashes were the result of the boat motor prop cutting through her leg as it went by. Her wounds were now bleeding profusely. "Let's get her out of the water," Kathy ordered.

We picked Mary up carefully and carried her to the grass. Kathy and I slapped large trauma dressings on her leg to try to stop the bleeding. We put pressure bandages on the deepest wounds.

I took over the injury that the Engine Three crew had been working on. There was an artery squirting blood, so I grabbed forceps and clamped the artery. That stopped the bleeding for now.

"Please get the stretcher from the Rescue," I said to the Engine Three crew. "We will transport." We applied pressure dressings to all the wounds and wrapped her whole leg with gauze. Her blood pressure was very low, at 100/40, and her pulse was too high: 120 BPM. From these readings, we knew she had lost a lot of blood. When the blood pressure is that low with injuries like these, it means her body did not have enough blood to push efficiently. The fast pulse rate was because her heart was trying to make up for the loss of blood.

I started an IV with Ringer's lactate and rolled the valve wide open. The Engine Three crew already had her on oxygen. "We'd better hurry," I said quietly, not wanting to excite the patient.

The stretcher was right beside us now. Once Mary was safely on it, we pushed her up the hill through the gate and into the back of our Rescue. Kathy and Bill were in back, and I drove again. They were busy attending to her wounds, so I called the hospital.

"West Bloomfield Fire Rescue Two to Blue Ridge Hospital, over."

"This is Blue Ridge Hospital, go ahead Rescue Two."

"We are inbound to your facility with a 22 year-old female that was run over by a speed boat prop while waterskiing. She has multiple deep U-shaped lacerations on her right leg and has lost a lot of blood," I continued.

"She had one arterial bleed which has a hemostat on. The bleeding has been controlled, but she is in shock. BP is 100/40 and pulse is 120 BPM. Respirations are about twenty and labored. The patient is cool and clammy. We have started an IV of Ringer's wide open. We need a surgery team standing by. It's difficult to tell how much blood she's lost because most of it was in the water. ETA about twelve minutes," I finished.

"Ok, Rescue Two, we will have a team standing by," the hospital confirmed. "Monitor her vitals and let us know if it changes."

"Ok, see you in about eleven minutes."

Lucky for her (and for us), her vitals improved a bit because of the Ringer's and the fact that we had stopped the bleeding. When we arrived at the hospital, there was a trauma team standing by. We wheeled her through emergency and directly into a trauma room. She was immediately given blood. The doctor removed the dressings on her wounds and exposed the open flesh. Some of the lacerations were clear to the bone, about one to two inches wide.

The ER doctor ordered her to be bandaged back up and sent to the operating room. And just like that she was gone. We did the paper work and headed back to the station.

"That will leave some scars," Kathy said.

"It will for sure," I agreed. "She probably has nerve damage. I hope it can be repaired in surgery," I added as Kathy reached for the mic.

She called in, "Rescue Two in service."

The dispatcher came back with, "That's good because you have another run at the public beach again. A possible choking victim. Time out, 1224. Be advised police are enroute."

"Rescue Two responding," Kathy called in the mic as she flipped on the emergency lights. We pulled onto a subdivision road to do a U-turn and go back the way we had come.

"What is it about that beach today?" I wondered out loud.

"I won't be going swimming there anytime soon," Kathy replied.

On hot summer days there were quite a few water accidents. We arrived in front of the gated fence at the same time as the police. We quickly retraced our steps back up the grassy hill and down to the sandy beach. A group of people were kneeling on the ground. One woman was jumping and waving her arms at us. The police officer, who turned out to be Miller, took some of our equipment so we could get there faster.

"She was eating a hotdog and it got stuck in her throat," yelled the middle aged woman. A seventy-two year old woman was sitting on the grass with her back supported against an oak tree. Her eyes were open and she looked at me with terror. She was not breathing. Then she passed out in front of us. I picked her up from behind and put my arms around her, locking my fist against her upper abdomen and quickly squeezed my arms to try to force the object out of her trachea. Nothing came out.

"Do it again!" Kathy yelled to me. I repeated the Heimlich maneuver with no success. The older woman's face was now blue and her body was relaxed. I knew that she was about to go into cardiac arrest, so I tried one more time.

This time I did it as hard as I could. Nothing. All the times I had practiced that maneuver I was good at it, so it was a surprise that it didn't work. We tried to pound her back to get it out. Nothing.

Kathy got out the cricoid kit and handed it to me. The cricoid stick was what we used when someone had a blocked airway. It was a last resort measure. We had tried everything else and wouldn't have much time before she would die. It doesn't matter what you do, if you can't get air to the patient, they die anyway.

I pushed the needle through the cricoid process into the trachea while drawing back on the syringe in order to create a vacuum. When I drew air into the syringe, I would know I'd reached the trachea. As
I pushed the needle deeper into her neck, I thought, "I should have gotten air by now."

All the times I had trained for this procedure, I was told it was an easy stick. But I wasn't getting anything. This was the first cricoid stick I or anyone else in the department had ever done.

"I should be in by now," I said, getting more alarmed. I pulled back harder on the syringe. I saw something brown fill the tube, then more brown.

"That's hotdog!" I yelled.

"Let's try lower," Kathy suggested.

"Ok, I'll try it lower." I pulled the syringe out and emptied it of the piece of hotdog. I tried again lower, below the cricoid. We were not supposed to go any lower than her Adam's apple, but I was never told what to do if the "crick stick" didn't work. It always worked, we were told. We didn't have anything to lose at this point, so I pushed the needle in again while drawing back the plunger. To our disbelief, I drew hotdog again.

"What the???" I called out as I removed the needle. "Let's try lower," I said in desperation.

A fairly large crowd had gathered behind us, and were getting restless. I again cleared the syringe of hotdog. I was going to try the lowest part of the trachea. So I put the needle in the neck, just above the sternum.

"Last chance," I murmured as I inserted the needle. I drew back on the syringe as I pushed the needle deeper. I was still getting resistance until I reached where the trachea was supposed to be. Then I drew in another piece of hotdog.

"$@!#*," Kathy cursed, as I pulled out the needle.

"Let's get her into the ambulance!" I yelled. The ambulance had just arrived with their stretcher. There was nothing more for us to do except transport. We put the lady on the stretcher and hooked her up to the LIFEPAK. The monitor showed her heart had gone into ventricular tachycardia, meaning her heart had stopped beating but still had electrical activity.

We began cardiac compressions, but by the time we reached the ambulance, the monitor showed systole (flat line). Kathy and Bill went with the patient to the hospital. As you might expect, she was pronounced dead on arrival.

On the way back to the station Kathy said, "How in the world did she get that whole hot dog down her trachea?"

"I don't know," I answered, shaking my head. "It was pretty astonishing."

To this day, I wonder how it happened.

"I thought I was doing something wrong when I didn't get any air, until I saw the hotdog," I said as we pulled into the station driveway.

"Rescue Two at quarters," Kathy announced.

"Rescue Two at quarters received." As we backed into the stall, I was met by the lieutenant. He told
me, "Stan at Station Four wants you to call him when you can."

"Thanks, Lieutenant," I said as I made my way to the phone. I called Station Four and Stan answered. He told me that Bugsy had been hit by a car and was gone. Not a good day.

I couldn't help thinking about when my old dog Mugsy had passed. I had arrived home after a long shift one day and found Wendy waiting for me at the door.

"Mugsy's not getting out of bed," she told me in a sad voice. Mugsy had been weak for a while now, and I'd been carrying him up and down the stairs. Until now, however, he'd been able to get around level ground on his own. When I checked on him, Mugsy was lying in his own mess. "I guess it's time to put him down," I declared, feeling weary and sad.

"I guess it is, but can you do it when I'm not here?" she pleaded. "Ok, I will call Terri." Terri was a veterinarian and the wife of a firefighter. When I got her on the phone, I told her the situation. She was very understanding.

"I will be over tomorrow," she promised.

"Thank you," I replied gratefully. I hung up the phone and Wendy looked at me with tears in her eyes. We went over to Mugsy's bed and sat with him for a long time. He tried to get up to go outside. He whined as I helped him up and to the door. He couldn't make it. He let loose with both ends.

We helped him back to his bed, and he cried as we laid him down. It is hard putting your dog to sleep, but letting him fall asleep in his own bed was less stressful for all of us.

I told Wendy, "That reminds me of a story that my parents would tell us kids. My dad came home after a long road trip, and my mother greeted him at the door saying, 'Welcome home. The kids are sick and the dog is dead.'"

Somehow that story hit a funny bone, and we both laughed. Still, the house seemed empty without old Mugsy

# Chapter 19 - Matters of the Heart

A typical day at Station Two involved frequent medical runs at area rest homes and visits to the Jewish Federation Apartments (JFA). Smoke investigations at JFA frequently turned out to be residents burning toast.

I learned that construction was starting on Station Five on Maple Road, east of Orchard Lake Road. That would become the new main station when it was finished.

After a few shifts with Station Two, my new team and I got used to each other. When you work with people for twenty-four hours at a time, you learn their strengths, weaknesses and quirks fairly quickly. We spent more time together then we did with our families.

Of course there were some people that couldn't seem to get along with any one. In my humble opinion, those people thought too much of themselves. The department had a few that were so stuck up you couldn't even talk to them. But those people were on Unit Two or the OFU (what each unit affectionately called the other), if you know what I mean.

As it happened, whenever there was something missing from the Engine or Rescue, or when something was messed up at the station, it always turned out to be because of Unit Two. That crew would blame it on Unit One, of course. However, for the most part, everyone got along.

People in the department loved to pull pranks on one another. One time when we were sleeping, one guy got up and took an IV bag filled with cold water, strung tubing up through the ceiling tiles and put the end over the target person. He set it on a timer for early morning. When the timer went off, the IV started dripping on the mark. The dripping was slow and soft so he didn't wake until he was soaking wet, and then he didn't know why he was wet. When he awoke, everyone was still asleep. No one ever admitted who did it.

Another prank was when Unit One put liquid dish soap in the dishwasher before shift change. When Unit Two started the dishwasher at lunch, it overflowed with bubbles and coated the entire kitchen floor. They never found out what had happened. It might have been me...

One time I did a small prank on the Chief. My third Chief of the department, Poppelreiter, was a friend of mine. We played softball together on the same team. Most of the guys were scared of the Chief because he seemed mean to them. He really was a good guy, though. One day there were seven of us working at Station One. We were all in the living room or at the kitchen table eating a snack. The Chief was taking a shower in the room next to the living room/kitchen.

I thought it would be funny if I took a pot of cold water and poured it on the Chief. When I got the pot out, the guys were laughing and saying that I didn't have the guts. I filled it with cold water and carried it to the shower room door.

"Don't do it!"

"You wouldn't dare!" they whispered as I opened the door.

"No! No! Don't!" they protested as I walked in. The Chief was singing in the shower, oblivious behind the curtain. As I lifted the pot above the curtain rod, I realized I could really get into trouble for this. However, it was too late to back out now. I poured the water over the Chief's head.

He screamed, "Ahhhhh!!!!!!" and grabbed at me through the curtain. He almost caught me, but his hand slipped off. I ran out the door as he stuck his head out around the curtain, seeing me as I ran out.

"Johnson! I'm going to kick your ass!" Then the door closed behind me as I sprinted into an empty living room.

To my right were the half-eaten snacks on plates that were still wobbling. Not a soul was left. They were all hiding somewhere in the apparatus room. The truth is the Chief liked the idea of being pranked on because it meant he was being treated like one of the guys.

Another run came in later on. "Station Three and Rescue Two, you have a possible drowning on Mirror Lake. 7654 Mirror Lake Road, which runs south off of Pontiac Trail. Time out, 1643."

The doors went up and we went out. I rode shot gun on the Rescue that day, and I knew where Mirror Lake was, so I navigated. It was a long run from Station Two to Mirror Lake, but Rescue One was out on a call, so we had to take it.

"Rescue Two responding," I said. I set the mic back in the holder on the dash board as I flipped on the emergency lights.

"Be advised Engine Three and Rescue Two, a patrol car is on the scene and reports that a swimmer is now missing."

"Message received dispatch," I answered. "I guess we'd better step it up," I said, although I knew we couldn't go much faster.

"Engine Three responding from Kroger's."

"Man that happens a lot," Marty commented. He was driving this time. He was right. It did happen a lot. And that's because Station Three was now a two-man station, which meant the crew would have to take the Engine to Kroger to shop for meals.

"We will probably get there around the same time as Engine Three," I said to Marty. And we did.

I picked up the mic and announced, "Rescue Two and Engine Three on the scene." The address was not hard to find because a patrol car was in front of the house. We parked in the driveway of a large three-story house with a huge green grassy yard and rock gardens. Marty and I, along with the Engine Three crew, carried the equipment around the house to a dock that stretched out into the lake.

A police officer was on the dock talking to three young men in their twenties. It was Officer Miller again. We frequently we ran into each other.

When Miller saw us approach, he briefed us. He said that these men just got off work doing construction and had decided to go for a swim. They all dove in off the end of the dock, but their friend didn't come back up.

One of the construction workers told us, "He's always pulling pranks on us, so we figured he was hiding to scare us. We knew he wouldn't go far, because his clothes are still here." He pointed to the pile of clothes on the grass just off the dock.

"How long has he been missing?" asked Marty.

"About ten minutes," answered the wet construction worker.

"I don't think he would fool around like this," said another worker. "Besides, he rode here with us in my car."

We were not prepared for a water rescue. WBFD did not have any equipment for that at the time. However, there was a rowboat tied to the dock. "Let's go out in the boat and see if we can spot him," I said, untying the rope that secured the boat.

"Should I call Oakland County?" Miller asked me.

I responded, "I guess you'd better. He is under the water until we find him somewhere else."

"Ok," Miller replied. "I will get Oakland County out here." He grabbed the mic that was on his uniform, and said into it, "Dispatch, we need Oakland County dive team out here ASAP."

"Ok, Eleven." Eleven is the number assigned to the police car that covered three's area. "I will call Oakland County dive team. It will take at least one half hour for them to get out to you."

"In the meantime, Marty and I will go out in the boat," I stated. "Why don't you three," I pointed to the construction workers, "go to the clump of trees over there and search."

I gave the co-workers of the missing man something to do so they would stay out of the way. We got in the boat and rowed off the end of the dock where he was last seen. We couldn't see anything below the water's surface. "Let's get the air mask off the Engine." Marty suggested.

"Good idea." I yelled to Bob, who was still on land, "Get just the face mask off the SCBA, ok?"

Bob nodded. In a few moments, he ran up to us with the face mask.

"Thanks, Bob," I said as he handed the mask to me.

I put the mask on then leaned over the side of the boat and put my face in the water. Marty rowed around the end of the dock as I searched under the surface of the water. Officer Miller directed us to the spot where the worker may have gone down, but the water was too murky and deep to see anything.

Oakland County arrived and we climbed out of the boat. They were already in their wet suits. Officer Miller told them the story and where the missing man may have gone under. The dive team put on their breathing apparatus and slipped under the water where we had been searching. Marty and I got the resuscitation equipment ready just in case.

About a minute later, one of the two divers poked his head out of the water and said, "We found him!" Then he slid back down beneath the water.

I got the intubation kit ready. The divers pushed the body out of the water and handed him to us. It took all five of us to get him onto the dock.

"It's cold down there," said a diver.

"That's good," I said. "Maybe he stands a chance."

He had been under water for forty-five minutes. In warm water he would stand no chance after that long. Just four or five minutes with no oxygen causes brain damage in most circumstances.

Kids have been known to survive for an hour under cold water. Hopefully it had been cold enough down there to keep this guy going. We laid him on the dock and started CPR with the bag mask. Marty could not get any air in.

"Let me intubate him," I said. I took the laryngoscope and looked into his throat. It was full of black muck and seaweed. I pulled out as much as I could before trying to stick the endotracheal tube in. Otherwise, the tube would go into his stomach.

I still could not see the vocal chords, so I took the esophageal tube out of the airway box and pushed it down his throat. The esophageal tube is supposed to go into the stomach and keep the contents from coming out and getting aspirated into the lungs. Then you can put the endotracheal tube in blind. Well, that was my theory any way.

I got the tube into the esophagus and then inserted the endotracheal tube into his mouth. I figured that it would have nowhere else to go but into the lungs. I had never heard of anyone doing that before, but it made sense to me.

I pushed the tube down his throat until I thought it was in far enough. I inflated the cuff, located around the bottom of the tube, with a syringe so it would not come out and no more junk would go into his lungs. Marty listened to his lungs while I bagged the patient.

"It's in!" Marty said excitedly, sounding surprised. "I didn't think that would work."

I bagged the patient while Bob did chest compressions. Marty hooked the patient up to the LIFEPAK, which showed an ECG of ventricular fibrillation.

Marty said, "Let's defibrillate him before I start the IV." Marty picked up the paddles and charged them to 100 Jules.

"Clear!" Marty called. I let go of the bag mask and Bob stopped compressions. Marty put the paddles on the patient's chest and pushed the buttons. The patient jumped as electricity coursed through him. We had to wait a few seconds for the monitor to go back to showing the ECG. There was no change.

"Continue CPR," I said as I started bagging the patient again. Bob went back to compressions.

"200 Jules!" Marty yelled. He reset the paddles and again put them on the patient's chest.

"Clear!" He discharged the paddles again, and the patient jumped. Again, there was no change.

"Trying 300!" Marty called. "Clear!" The LIFEPAK discharged again. There was still no change. We might have called it quits then, but because he was so young, only twenty-two, we kept working on him until we got to the hospital. We started an IV and administered drugs to try to start his heart, but nothing worked. When we arrived at the hospital, it did not take long for the ER doctor to call it.

"How long has he been without a heartbeat?" the doctor asked. "About an hour," I answered. "He was under water for forty minutes and we worked at the scene for ten minutes, then for the ten minutes to get here."

"Ok," The doctor said. "Time of death…" he looked up at the clock, "let's say five fifty-five."

We all stopped working on the patient and moved away. I took one look back before I went out the door. He was lying on the hospital gurney, tubes in his mouth and his arm. His eyes were wide open and were starting to dry out. I walked away, disappointed that we weren't able to save him.

What we think happened was that the construction workers decided to go for a swim after a long hot work day. The victim jumped into the water and went down deep. The shock of quickly going from extreme hot to extreme cold caused him to pass out. He was in good physical shape, so he sank to the bottom. Fat floats, muscle sinks. In the movies and on TV, the patient is always saved. But in real life, that doesn't happen too often.

It was my turn to do all of the paper work, like I've done a thousand times before. On a cardiac arrest, we administer a lot of drugs and each drug has to be written down. It takes a lot of time to complete the report. We try to document details as we go, but we don't always have time to record everything. The report I had to complete at the hospital was the Oakland County medical report. The ER required a copy of it. I also had to fill out a drug report, which was needed to replace our supply at the hospital pharmacy.

When we returned to the station, I had to finish the paper work and put it in the computer. Then there is a state incident report to be completed, followed by a blue station report. All of them had to be entered into the computer.

When I finally finished, it was 1930 hours. We had to get the dinner we had missed out of the refrigerator. After dinner we had to wash our dishes before we could relax. Then the tones went off.

"Station Two, you have a man down at 4522 Jefferson, which runs south off of Maple."

I felt heart burn flare up, and I burped as I headed to the watch desk. The lieutenant, Kathy, Marty and I went to the large wall map, then got the section map out of the drawer.

"We will take the Engine and Rescue," stated the lieutenant. We always had at least four people on a possible cardiac arrest.

I pulled the Rescue out first, and the Engine followed. Jefferson was in a subdivision that ran south off of Maple. It was a winding, low-traffic road with a lot of bikes, children and joggers.

As we came to a stop, I saw a small crowd of people. A bicyclist sat on his bike, wearing tight black riding shorts and a green tear-drop-shaped helmet next to a man of about fifty years old, who was lying on the side of the road.

"Rescue Two and Engine Two on scene," I said into the mic before climbing out. I was already getting out the equipment when I heard, "On scene received, Rescue Two and Engine Two."

Marty and I approached the older gentleman, who was wearing workout clothes. Someone said he had been jogging when he collapsed. Marty and I could see at a glance that he was in cardiac arrest. His eyes were open, and from his head to his nipple line was purple. Without saying anything to one another, we got to work.

We knew our job by the position we were in. I was at the head, so I took the airway. He was at the other side, so he took the quick-look paddles off the LIFEPAK and placed them on his chest. He held them still to see the monitor. The man was in V-fib.

"I'm going to charge the paddles," Marty announced. The quick-look paddles and the defibrillation paddles were the same thing. You can shock with them, but you can also use them to get a basic ECG.

"I'll start at 200 Jules," Marty said, setting the LIFEPAK accordingly. He pushed the charge button. I checked for a pulse, even though I knew there wasn't one. The worst thing we could do is defibrillate someone when they are not in arrest.

When the LIFEPAK was charged, Marty placed the paddles on the patient's chest and yelled, "Clear!" The defibrillator discharged, sending the man lurching. The monitor showed he was still in V-fib.

"Again!" I called out. Marty repeated the procedure.

"Clear!" He defibrillated the patient, but the monitor showed that nothing had changed.

"300 Jules!" Marty called out. "Clear!" He released the shock, making the man's whole body jump once more. Nothing changed.

"Ok," I said, "let's start CPR." The lieutenant started chest compressions as I prepared to intubate the patient. I looked in his mouth with the laryngoscope and saw vomit in his mouth and throat. I couldn't allow that to get into his lungs or he would not survive. I also couldn't see where to put the tube.

"Suction please," I forced myself to slow down, knowing I needed to stay in control of the situation. A life-threatening medical emergency can be overwhelming if we don't remain calm.

Someone handed me the suction catheter and I put it in his mouth. I placed my finger over the hole to make a suction. "Hisssssss." The sound let me know we had suction, and I was able to clear the throat of his thrown-up dinner.

"Now I can see the chords," I said to myself, inserting the tube between the vocal chords and inflating the syringe. Marty listened to his lungs while I squeezed the bag mask.

"It's in!" he called out. "You are two-for-two today." I handed the bag mask to Kathy, who was the engineer for this shift. She started bagging the patient.

"Survey the situation," I reminded myself. "Stand back. What's already done and what needs to be done? I have Kathy on the airway and Lt. Dale is on the chest. Marty has the LIFEPAK."

I pushed myself to think clearly and logically. "What needs to be done is to start an IV and to administer the proper drugs."

I got ready to start an IV. I looked for a vein in his arm, but could not see anything. I put a rubber tourniquet tight on his bicep, but no vein popped out. This was not a good time for his veins to hide. I felt for his brachial veins on both his arms and checked his hands. Nothing. I stuck the needle in where the brachial vein in his arm should be and hoped.

Hope doesn't usually start an IV, but in this case, it did. To my great surprise and relief, I got a blood flash in the syringe. I pushed in the drugs that protocol dictated at that time. I can't remember exactly what they were, because it changed over the years.

For instance, I know that I gave two fifty cc amps of sodium bicarbonate to start. That procedure changed later in my career, as many of them did. For example, we used to give calcium chloride as a last resort, but then we learned that it stops the heart. In fact, Michigan's own Doctor Kevorkian, aka "Doctor Death," used calcium chloride to stop his patients' hearts.

I followed the sodium bicarb with epinephrine. "Defibrillate again," I commanded. Marty charged the LIFEPAK to 300 Jules and shouted, "Clear!"

"Thump!" was the sound of the energy going from the machine into the patient. Again, there was no change. I had the clipboard to record the times everything was done and the names of drugs given to the patient.

After about ten defibs, it was time to transport to the hospital. Marty and I went with the patient in the ambulance. I called the hospital on the medical radio. I told the doctor what we had given the patient and that nothing had worked.

I was ordered by Dr. Schmart to do an intracardiac injection and then to defibrillate again. I had never done that before. To my knowledge, no one else in the department had done it either. We did carry a syringe for that procedure with us. It had a three-inch long needle.

I took it out of the drug box and pulled the cap off. I pushed the air out of the syringe, followed by a small squirt of liquid. By this point, we were well on the way to the hospital. I counted the patient's ribs, starting at his clavicle, down five on the left side of his sternum. I felt the space between the fifth and sixth rib with my finger. I
pushed the three inch needle into his chest next to my finger while drawing back on the plunger like I did with the cricoid stick.

This time, when I reached the heart, I would know I was in by drawing blood into the syringe rather than air. I only hoped it would go better than it had with the cricoid stick. I pushed the needle farther into his chest and drew back the plunger. Blood backed up into the syringe. I was in the heart.

I pushed the large dose of epinephrine from the syringe into his heart and then removed the needle. I put the cap back on and threw the syringe into the sharps container.

"Ok," I said. "Defibrillate again." Marty defibrillated the patient, and it worked. The patient was in a cardiac ventricular rhythm. Not a good rhythm, but he had a pulse. The danger of giving an intracardiac injection is if you inject the epinephrine into the heart tissue you will cause terminal ventricular fibrillation, which means you've killed him.

You might hit a cardiac artery and give him another heart attack. You might miss the heart all together. Anyway, I got it and it worked. The patient remained unconscious, though. When we turned him over to the ER staff, they continued to work on him. Unfortunately, he didn't survive.

Bob, from Station Three, philosophized, saying, "He was a jogger. He used up all his heart beats. You only have so many in your life, so don't use them up."

That's one way to justify not exercising, I guess.

When we got back to the station, guess who was waiting for me? It was my favorite, Captain Slasher.

He sneered sarcastically, "Johnson you really want to get into trouble, don't you?"

"What did I do now?"

"You know that you need to stop the ambulance and pull to the side of the road when you give an intracardiac injection," he chastised me like a child.

"I was successful," I pointed out.

"It doesn't matter that you were successful," he admonished. "It matters what I say." He turned and walked out.

"That's what I call an 'at-ah-boy,'" I commented in frustration.

There's nothing like getting chastised for doing your job well.

# Chapter 20 - The Power of Horses

I always tried to keep busy on my days off. An old friend of mine owned a small ambulance company, Huron Valley Ambulance, based in Highland (not to be confused with HVA in Ann Arbor). He asked me to work the ambulance for the games at the Detroit Polo Club out there. Since it was a good way to make a little extra cash, I agreed.

I would work with a paramedic named Jack. We met at the small garage where the ambulance was housed the morning of the game. Jack drove the vehicle to the polo grounds.

"This is a good way to make easy money," Jack assured me. "You just kick back and watch a polo match." Jack had worked with AVA for a long time. He was doing this as a side job as well.

We pulled the rig onto the dirt parking lot and parked it by the gate. The playing surface for polo was a green grassy football field-sized arena. Each end had goal uprights as well. The whole thing was enclosed by a long white wooden fence. We entered through a white gate and headed towards the stands.

The manager met us there and said, "We've never had a problem here, apart from a few minor accidents. So find yourselves a seat, relax and enjoy the match."

People filed into the stands. The riders led their horses one after another towards the field. The smell of popcorn and cigar smoke perfumed the air.

I kept the first aid kit between my feet, under the green wooden chair. There was not a cloud in the blue sky. A brisk breeze blew my hair into my eyes. The sweat rolling off my forehead quickly evaporated in the steady wind.

About a half hour later, the stands were full of excited fans. The white ball was dropped and the match began. It was amazing that the horses seemed to follow the ball. The riders smashed the ball with their mallets while the horses ran right at one another other, barely avoiding colliding each time.

The horses kicked grass clumps into the air as they ran. Clouds of dust followed the horses. I reached down to get my first handful of popcorn. I looked up as I tipped the popcorn into my mouth. Time seemed to slow down

as I watched two horses collide head-on. One horse somersaulted across the field, his rider vaulting into the air
over it. Horse and rider fell to the ground in a cloud of dust and grass clumps.

The second horse ran a few more steps before collapsing. It was hard to see through the dust at first. The stands were silent, still and stunned. We all held our breath, waiting to see if everyone was all right. The first horse and the rider got up right away. The second horse was on his side, kicking violently into the air. I looked for
the other rider. After the dust cleared away in the wind, I saw him trapped under the kicking horse. He was motionless.

Although this all took only a few seconds, it seemed longer. Jack yelled to me, "You go to the rider and I'll get the ambulance!"

I snatched the first aid kit and raced to the horse and rider in the middle of the field. Blood was now pouring out of the horse's nostrils, each breath blowing red droplets into the air. The rider's right leg was pinned under the horse, which had finally stopped kicking.

I assessed the man's condition. He was unconscious, but still breathing. Blood from the horse was showering down and covering us like red rain. Jack pulled the ambulance up to the mess and got out the stretcher and the long back board. The rider, still trapped under the horse, had a fractured femur.

Jack joined me as we tried to figure out how we were going to get the patient out from under the injured animal. There were likely spinal injuries in addition to the fracture. So, how to get him out without injuring him further? Meanwhile the horse was still blowing great amounts of blood into the air.

The first thing we did was put a cervical collar on the patient. The question of how to get the horse off the patient was decided for us. A mob emerged from the stands, screaming and heading toward us. We tried to warn them that the patient had to be put on a back board, but the crowd wasn't listening or rational.

They overwhelmed us and pulled on the horse and the rider. Jack and I tried to stop them from injuring the patient further, but we were no longer in control. Some of the mob grabbed Jack and I and held us back as the wild crowd seized the patient under the arms and jerked him out from under the horse. They picked up the rider and carried him to the ambulance. Someone else pushed the stretcher. Once everything was in the ambulance, they let us go. I'd had never seen anything like that pandemonium before or since.

We got into the vehicle and started to pull away when I heard a gunshot. "They must have put the horse down," I thought to myself. I turned my thoughts back to the patient. I could see the femur bone bulging against the skin on his thigh, nearly ready to break through. Jack turned on the emergency lights and siren as we sped towards the hospital. I put a traction splint on his leg, which insured that the femur bone would not break through the skin. I checked the rest of the patient for other injuries.

He had a number of evolutions, or v-shaped lacerations, on his arms and leg that would need stitches, so I bandaged the wounds. I took his shoes off and was checking his feet to assess spinal injury when he said, "What happened? Where am I?"

"You were playing polo and had an accident," I answered.

"How is my horse?" he asked right away, clearly more concerned about the animal than himself at that moment.

"Right now let's concentrate on you," I said to distract him. "Can you move your legs?" I needed to assess his spinal condition but I also thought it would be best for him to not think of his horse right now. He wasn't having any of it.

"Tell me how my horse is!" he insisted.

I paused for a moment and said, "I'm sorry, but I don't think he made it." He didn't say a word when he wiggled his feet.

Then he asked, "What happened?"

He repeated that question every minute or two all the way to the hospital, forgetting that I had already explained. That told me that he had a closed head injury. When patients are in significant accidents that may involve a head injury they can experience short-term memory loss. He probably would not remember me or the accident at all.

I read about the accident the next day in the paper. The rest of the polo match was cancelled, and the rider would make a full recovery. It didn't say the crowd could have paralyzed or killed him. It was astonishing that he wasn't injured more than he was. That was my last ride with HVA Highland, since they went out of business shortly after that run.

The next day, at Station Two, I came in at 0730 hours. I was sitting at the kitchen table drinking coffee and talking with the four Unit Two boys when Kathy, Bill and lieutenant arrived. The guys had just been telling me about the Silver Cook Condominiums on Maple, east of Haggerty Road. Lieutenant Rick had apparently told them, "Be aware that the builder of those condos did not follow proper electrical code. They used aluminum wiring instead of copper."

Aluminum wire was used for wiring in houses for a short time, but it was found to get hot quickly because it doesn't conduct electricity as well as copper. It fails when it gets hot and can cause a fire.

I agreed to cover for one of the guys so he could leave early. I was now officially on duty. And then, of course, the tones immediately went off. "Station Two. You have a medical at Jewish Federation Apartments, apartment 4543. Patient fell down and can't get up. Time out, 0735."

Luckily for me, I was working for the lieutenant, so I was scheduled to be on the Engine. I stayed at the table drinking coffee while the OFU went to the Rescue on what we called a "Gomer run." These were basically nonlife-threatening calls from rest homes that ate up time and resources. We had a large amount of Gomer runs to those apartments.

Sometimes it's nice staying back when a run comes in. Being on the Rescue, you are always on a medical at Station Two. It only took about fifteen minutes for them to put the patient back on her chair, but that was an extra half hour I had to relax and settle in.

One thing that we did a lot was pick up residents of the Federation Apartments. I mean literally pick them up off the floor, even if they had slid softly and were uninjured. The staff there would not get the resident up and would not let the individual get up themselves. We would have to go over there and pick them up. The Apartments advertise that they offer a full medical staff, but what they didn't say is that it's really the WBFD caring for their residents.

At 0800 hours, the Rescue was back on duty. I was assigned to ride shot gun, Kathy was driving and Bill was on the Engine. We also had a new rookie, or subby, that had started the previous month. The subby was on watch duty and rode third on the Engine.

We had a few Gomer runs during the day, but nothing too exciting happened. After dinner we settled down in front of the TV. I was going to lift weights after the food settled, but as Bill and I got ready to exercise, the tones went off.

"Station Two. You have a PIA in the intersection of Orchard Lake Road and Fourteen Mile. Time out, 2138."

We climbed into the vehicles and drove out the door. It was dark, so the lights bounced off the side of the fire station and the road as we pulled onto Maple. Rescue Two was in the lead, followed by Engine Two.

"Engine Two and Rescue enroute to Orchard Lake and Fourteen Mile," the lieutenant called in. Maple Road was also called Fifteen Mile. Fourteen Mile was a mile south from that, which put the PIA only three miles away from the station. Three minutes later we called in on scene.

"At the scene received, Engine Two. Be advised, I have a patrol car on the way. ETA about two minutes."

We pulled up to the intersection, seeing smoke billowing up from a large semi-truck, facing us with her four-way signals flashing. A man came out from behind the truck and waved his arms to get our attention. There was a lot of traffic out for 9:30 p.m., and the cars were not slowing down despite the crash. Usually, traffic slows
because of gawking, but not these people. They were clearly too busy to bother.

We pulled the Rescue beside the rear of the semi-trailer. The man was still jumping up and down and pointing at the back of the rig. I flipped on the switch that turned on the side spot lights mounted on the vehicle. The scene was drenched in bright light. Now we could see the rear end of a new-looking black Corvette, with its lights still on. The front had disappeared under the trailer. There were black and white pieces of fiberglass scattered around the scene. Corvettes are made of fiberglass, so I knew the debris was from that car.

It looked as though the front had exploded, sending scattered pieces in all directions. I got out with my clipboard and went around the side sticking out into the traffic. I took the orange trauma kit from Bill. When I turned to get around the Rescue, the box was ripped from my grip by a car hitting it and just missing me. The driver had been gawking at the accident and nearly took me out in the process!

A police officer on the scene yelled at the driver, but the car did not slow. The officer hit the car with his black foot-long flashlight, putting a large dent in the fender as it sped away.

Luckily the trauma box was not damaged and had stayed shut. Having that thing pop open and dumping the hundreds of bandages and gauze pads and other objects all over the place would have been a disaster. I had already experienced that before, and was glad it wasn't repeated this night.

I picked up the trauma box as the police officer asked me, "Are you all right?"

I brushed off, saying, "He missed me, but it was a nice try."

We made our way to the Corvette. I stumbled over a hubcap that was lying on the road. It couldn't have been from the Corvette because those cars don't have hubcaps. As we approached, the officer shone his flashlight into the part of the Corvette that was jammed under the trailer. Every semi now has a rear underride guard installed on the back in order to stop a vehicle from passing under it. Well, this one had failed, and now lay useless on the pavement.

Behind the steering wheel was the driver's body. I could only see the torso sitting straight up, covered in a large amount of blood that had run down the chest, pooling on both the seat and the floor.

"OH MY GOSH! LOOK AT THAT! LOOK AT THAT!" yelled a hysterical voice from behind me. In surprise, I glanced back. The rookie's face was pale, his eyes wide open and pointing to the back of the Corvette. Behind the driver's seat was a set of eyes looking straight at me, locked in a look of terror. The eyes looked out from a head that was splattered with blood. The neck was not attached to anything. It had been a clean cut.

It was very eerie, seeing a dismembered head lying behind the seat, looking directly at me. The rookie began dry heaving, and slapped his hand over his mouth. He ran, doubled over, to the side of the road, where I heard more loud gagging noises. Bill and I smile knowingly at one another briefly before we got to work.

Obviously the driver was dead, but was there anyone else in there? I crawled under the trailer to the other side of the Corvette to see if anyone was trapped. Luckily there wasn't. I was kneeling in sticky green engine coolant, feeling it soak into my pants.

We learned that the semi had stopped at a red light and the Corvette had slammed into the back of the trailer, decapitating the driver clean as a whistle and depositing his head in the back area. The guard that was supposed to prevent exactly this from happening had been too weak and broke off when the Corvette hit it.

The driver of the semi was sitting in a patrol car, crying as he was questioned. When I first started in the Department, semi-trailers did not have underride guards at the back, so we had a lot of K's (kills) from rear impacts. This was the first K caused by such a crash that I'd seen since the law had taken effect.

"I guess you should call the ME," I said to Officer Miller. "I already did," he said, staring at the corpse.

"He had pretty eyes," I heard Rich say from next to me.

Then I replied, "He's got his father's eyes." Rich smiled, but Officer Miller just shook his head. He knew we were just lightening the mood, or maybe he thought we were really crazy.

It dawned on me that Rich hadn't been here earlier. "What are you doing here?" I asked him.

"The lieutenant at Station One thought you guys might need help, so I came over in the pickup," he answered. "But I guess there is nothing left to do but pick up the pieces. I guess I will 'head' back," he added.

Just as he was climbing into Utility One, Rich turned to me and yelled, "Don't lose your head. You know, he had to head off to work. Maybe he was just trying to get too far ahead." Then he got in the cab and drove off. It was my turn to shake my head, thankful it was still attached. I began completing the paperwork. This incident took a lot of time to write up.

I was present when the wrecker pulled out what was left of the Corvette from under the semi. I saw the ME arrive in the meat wagon, take out his stretcher and, with the help of two ambulance crew, put the dead driver in a body bag. He placed the head in a
separate bag and set it on the stretcher. Finally he wheeled the driver
to the ambulance.

The ambulance left, lights flashing. That seemed odd since in this situation, there was no hurry. The wrecker winched the mangled car onto its bed and left.

Engine Two used the two and a half inch hose to spray the engine fluids, and whatever else was left, off the road. Then they packed up the hose and went back to the station. As I finished up my report, Officer Miller came up to me with a cell phone. He lifted it in the air and said, "Apparently, the driver was texting."

# Chapter 21 - Heroics; Fighting Fires and Saving Cats

After we returned to the station, we put the Engine and Rescue back together, and I went to take a shower. I wanted to wash off the engine coolant that had soaked through to my leg, as well as the blood that inevitably got on me. The tones went off again as I was drying myself with a towel.

"Station Two, Station One, Station Three." When dispatch named three stations, it meant a structure fire. Sure enough. "You have a structure fire at 3478 Silver Cook Lane, in the Silver Cook Condos. I've had several calls saying smoke is coming out of the eaves. Time out, 2300."

I rushed to put my clothes on. Do you have any idea how difficult it is to put your clothes on when you're wet and in a hurry? I put on shorts and a tee shirt, my bunker gear and fire coat and I was ready to go.

The lieutenant had already looked up the best route to get there by the time I got to the watch desk. "Engine Two will stretch from the hydrant to the front of the condo," the lieutenant commanded as we made our way to the trucks. "Rescue will be attack."

"Engine Two, Rescue Two responding," the lieutenant called on the radio as we pulled out of the apparatus room doors.

"Engine Two and Rescue Two responding received," dispatch answered.

I was in the back of the Rescue putting my SCBA on. Kathy was driving, and the new rookie was in the back of the Engine. The lieutenant rode shotgun on the Engine and Bill drove.

"Engine One, Rescue One, Ladder One and Captain's car responding," the Captain called.

"Engine Three, Tanker Three responding," said a voice over the radio. "Responding received Engine One, Rescue One, Ladder One, Captain's Car, Engine Three, Tanker Three. At 2301 hours."

There is always a lot of traffic on the radio during a major structure fire. We pulled out behind the Engine heading west on Maple Road. As we rushed to the fire, I finished strapping on my SCBA equipment. One strap went over my right shoulder, the other strap over my left shoulder. Then I had to click the straps together across my chest. I felt the forty-pound carbon fiber air tank resting on my back. Before, they had been made of steel. I buckled the waist strap and tightened it as we turned north onto Silver Cook Lane.

I knew we were almost there, so I quickly put the mask on, making sure it was a good fit. I tested the seal by covering the end of the rubber tube leading to the air tank with my hand and breathing in to make a suction. No air was getting into my mask, so it passed the test.

I attached the tube to my air tank and opened the regulator by twisting the knob. Cool air rushed into the mask so I could breathe. Then, as I was putting my helmet on, the Rescue turned and I lost my balance for a moment. I slammed into the side of the truck. I righted myself as we came to a stop.

"Station Two on scene, reporting a two-story attached condo with flames coming out of the lower windows. Two condos now involved and eight others are at risk." I didn't hear the dispatcher's responses as I was jumping out of the back of the Rescue. My heart was pounding as I went to the Engine to help pull the two and a half cross lays.

The lieutenant stood, silhouetted in front of the blaze, and ordered, "Pull both cross lays to the front of the condo!" I took the rookie with me to the other side of the Engine to pull out the second cross lay. I took my mask off, letting it hang down by the strap. I shut down the air from the tank to save it for later.

I grabbed the hose sticking out of what we called ears and pulled as hard as I could. With the extra adrenaline I had, the line came out all at once and slid to the pavement with a plop. I ordered the rookie to take the nozzle and drag the hose around the front of the Engine to the condo. The hose was flat and light when there's no water in it, so he could do it alone.

I straightened out all the kinks and then pulled the rest of the one hundred and fifty foot long hose around the Engine to the fire. The first cross lays were already out and straightened, all ready to be charged.

As we got our second line ready, I heard sirens close by. The Ladder truck was arriving, lights flashing and sirens blaring. Kathy and I went to the lawn area of the condo next to the one that was on fire.

The lieutenant told us, "Go in and don't let the fire get into this residence." We nodded our heads as we fit the masks to our faces and turned the air back on. The bell rang on the air tank, indicating that our masks were charged and ready to go.

Bill, the engineer, pulled the lever on the side of the Engine, sending water into our hoses. The water pressure caused the hose to writhe like a snake as it filled. When the water reached the nozzle, it began pouring out until I shut it down.

The other hose was lying in front of the residence that was on fire. Even with my mask on, I could smell the odor of smoke that was starting to gather around us. Engine One and Rescue One, followed by Ladder One, pulled up behind us. The lieutenant signaled for us to go in.

With the nozzle in my left hand and Kathy behind me, I grabbed the door knob. The door was locked. The lieutenant pointed, so I kicked the door open. We entered the condo's front room. I could see a little, but the smoke was getting thicker, and it was beginning to get hotter. Kathy and I went down to our knees where it was cooler.

My face mask became cloudy, so I wiped my gloved hand across the Plexiglas and cleared the wet soot that had already gathered. For a while, I could see somewhat better. We crawled ahead in the direction of the fire.

I could hear the chattering from the hand radio that was in the front top pocket of my turn-out coat. Kathy said something to me, but I couldn't understand her through all the gear. We pressed ahead to a large living room. I could see a red glow on the ceiling. I opened the nozzle and sprayed it with a powerful blast of water, which rebounded off the wall and back onto us.

The red lightened in color, but not for long. When it came back, it was even stronger. I could see flames heading for us, so I opened the nozzle and blasted them with a powerful stream of water. The flames only got bigger and hotter. I turned my head to Kathy and yelled, "We have to back up."

She shouted back, "Maybe we should get out." I desperately sprayed the fire while backtracking. We heard some noise over the radio. "Rescue Two! Rescue Two! Get out! Get out! Get out now!"

I backed up faster, pushing Kathy behind me. We realized that the roof may come down at any time. We couldn't see at all now. The condo was full of black smoke. We could feel and hear small pieces of ceiling bouncing off our helmets and coats. We followed the hose line backward, and the ceiling crashed to the floor right where we had just been. A blast of air blew past our head, peppering us with hot embers that banged off my face mask and chest. I kept the hose trained on the raging hungry fire as it chased us out.

We reached the front door, which was held open for us by the rookie. The lieutenant stood right next to him. Kathy and I backed out the door, smoke following us in a cloud that rose up into the sky. As I got up to my feet, black ashes fell off my helmet onto the concrete porch.

We stepped off the porch, where the lieutenant met us and pointed to the rest area that had been set up. The rookie brushed away the still-glowing embers that had landed on my shoulder. I removed the mask from my face, and only then realized that my low- air alarm bell had been ringing. I reached back and turned off the air.

At the rest area, I took my helmet from my head and set it on the tarp that had been laid out. Someone helped me pull the SCBA tank off my back, which helped. Kathy and I rested for a while as we surveyed the current scene.

The Ladder truck was parked in front of the condo complex, the bucket extended to the roof. From the bucket, a four-inch hose and nozzle sprayed huge amounts of water on the raging fire that was now through the roof of both condos.

We were in danger of losing the all ten residences. There were about six firefighters spraying water into the lower part of the condo and four men on the roof, cutting holes to ventilate it. Extension ladders stretched against the building up to the roof.

Our team was trying to get ahead of the fire, but it was moving too fast. "With the fire stops built into the attics, it shouldn't be moving that quickly," I said to Kathy.

The Chief had arrived and was running the show. He had been notified of the fire and had come in from home. The fire stretched high into the black smoke-filled sky. Glowing embers shot up with the soot, disappearing into the night. Some of the hot embers floated back down, little red lights that landed all around us before going out. I took a drink of water from the plastic bottle that someone had handed to me.

I was watching the firefighters working on the burning roof when I saw a man fall through. After a moment, he managed to pull himself back up. Over the radio I heard, "Get off the roof! Get them off the roof! Ladder One, extend the ladder to the men and get them off!" That was the Chief himself giving those orders. He had obviously seen what I had just seen.

The Ladder truck turned the ladder towards the condo where the firefighters were and extended it to the roof. The bucket rested on the edge of the roof and the four men climbed in. The ladder retracted back toward the Engine and then the ground.

I heard a crash. When I looked back to the roof where these men had just been standing moments ago, I saw it collapse into itself. It seemed to happen in slow motion, as it sank into the building and out of sight. A large plume of fire, ash, smoke and superheated gasses exploded into the air and disappeared into the dark. That had been a close call.

Kathy and I, recovered from our efforts, were ready to get back to work. We put on a fresh SCBA tank and prepared to head back to the fire for assignment. We finished gearing up just as the firefighters that had escaped the roof reached the recovery area.

"I'm glad you guys got off of there. You had me worried for a minute," I said to them. The guys plopped down on the tarp, exhausted. Kathy and I helped them get their air tanks off and then gave them bottles of water. Other people were there to help also. There were several volunteers bringing us drinks, coffee and food.

When we returned to the inferno, the lieutenant waved us toward him. "I need you to go in and help Dan upstairs. He's putting out a small fire up there," he said to me. Then he added, "And Kathy, I need you on another project."

She stayed with the lieutenant to get her orders while I put on my air mask again. I tightened the straps on my head, which also pulled my hair back. I replaced my helmet, turned on my air tank and headed upstairs.

When I reached the top of the stairs, I heard yelling. Dan was alone and had fallen through the floor. Fortunately, he had caught himself with his arms out. There was smoke coming out of the hole that he had made. Because of that, I figured there must be fire below him. "Get me the hell out of here!" he yelled.

He was about five feet away from a wall and ten feet from me. The floor was weak, spongy and sloped, funneling down to the hole. There was a lot of debris scattered all around him. Sharp objects, like nails, were embedded in the broken pieces of wood lying about. I knew that if I walked to him, I would probably fall in too.

Instead, I lay down on the floor, facing Dan. I stretched out as long as I could, spreading my weight across as much area as possible. I inched toward him, trying to be cautious for both our sakes. When I finally reached him, I grabbed his gloved hand and tried to pull him up.

He moved slightly, so I knew I should be able to pull him out. Knowing he was probably scared, I *tried* to lighten the mood and said, "If you go, we both go." That was a quote from the movie *Backdraft*. He didn't get the reference, so I let it go.

I pulled him out a little at a time. He was able to use my arm to pull himself up further. About ten minutes of effort finally freed him from the floor that had nearly swallowed him. We both crawled back to solid floor.

Over the years, Dan would often bring that experience up when we got together. Sharing such a traumatic incident connects people in a very unique way.

Once free of the hole, we both left the building. Dan went to the rest center while I went back to the fire. I was stood next to Kathy at the front of the condo that was just ahead of the fire. A resident screamed at us, "My cat! My cat, Fluffy, is in there!"

"Ma'am, get back," the lieutenant called to her, "we will do what we can to get your cat, but you have to get back for your safety." As she backed away, she said, "Fluffy is my whole life."

At that moment, a news camera and microphone was stuck in my face. The reporter asked me a question that I couldn't understand. The gear and the noise at the scene simply made hearing a challenge. Instead of answering, I pointed to my right where the Chief was standing. The lieutenant did the same. The reporter nodded and headed toward the Chief. "Go in and see if you can find that damn cat," the lieutenant ordered.

"Ok, Lieutenant," I said, putting my mask on again. As I prepared to go in, I noticed the fire was a little less intense. It looked like we were finally getting a handle on it.

Kathy and I turned on our flashlights, opened the unlocked door and went inside. It was not very hot in there, with only a light cloud of smoke hanging in the air. I could see well enough with my flashlight to navigate around the condo. We looked in each room one by one. In the bedroom, under a bed, we found a set of bright green eyes reflecting back at us.

"I found the cat," I said. In addition to the cat, we were searching for anyone else who might be trapped in the condo. Now that we had found the animal, we had to catch it. That was a different proposition altogether. I went to the far side of the bed and Kathy stayed on the near side. I made noise as I positioned myself, trying to spook the cat out. When I reached under the bed, Fluffy meowed in fear and ran straight to Kathy.

She caught it and yelled, "Got him!"

"Kathy," I said, "You take the cat to its owner. You be the hero." "No, you take it," Kathy replied. "I have something I want to check out. There might be another animal here. I found some kind of cage," she claimed.

"Ok," I relented. I scooped up the cat and walked out with the squirming furball in my arms. As I looked for the owner, there was a bright flash, which blinded me for a moment. As my eye sight returned, I found a reporter in front of me, taking my picture. "Great," I said to myself, "that's just what I need. A picture of me and a cat."

The guys would have a good laugh if that picture was published in the paper. I quickly put that out of my mind as I spotted the owner. She came running up to me and grabbed the cat out of my arms and hugged and kissed it. Then she turned to me and said "Thank you so, so much for saving my Fluffy!"

"You're welcome. Just doing my job," I responded, a bit embarrassed. "I have to get back to work."

It wasn't much of a rescue. In my opinion, I had better things to do then search for a stupid cat. Now if it had been a dog...

By this time the sun was up and the fire was mostly out. Kathy and I helped put out the rest of the small fires. I went back upstairs with an inch and a half hose, adjusted the nozzle and sprayed a straight stream on the smaller fire that was burning in a back room. The water hit the flames and the sheer force of the stream quickly knocked it down and scattered the embers and debris that was around the area. I sprayed that whole room and the rest of the place before leaving.

By that time it was after 0800. The lieutenant approached us said, "You have been relieved by the OFU. Let's go home."

We were all exhausted. It was about 9:30 when I finally got home, and I hadn't slept a wink during my whole shift. Maybe that's how I ended up sleeping the whole day and the night away, too.

# Chapter 22 - A Good Day At the Office

In my younger years, I had been a full-contact kick boxer, which was the predecessor to the UFC, or cage fighting. The day after I earned my brown belt in Koei Kan Karate, I was in the locker room getting my gi on when I heard a commotion in the dojo. I couldn't see what was going on, but soon enough I learned that a cocky young man wanted to take on someone from our school. Sounds stupid, I know, but true.

Once I was ready, I walked out into the practice area. It was thirty feet by thirty feet, with long vertical mirrors lining the walls. The floor was covered with mats, and there were swords and other martial arts weapons displayed above the mirrors.

As I stepped on the mat, I noticed a man talking to my Sensei, or teacher. "Mr. Johnson!" my Sensei called to me. He always called everyone "mister."

"Get ready to spar," he directed, indicating that he wanted me to fight the man he had been talking with. I had no idea what was going on, but I stretched out and was soon ready. Sensei gave us boxing gloves and sparring masks to put on. The guy, whom I didn't recognize, refused his mask, so I did too. We faced off in the middle of the room.

The Sensei asked, "Ready?" We both shook our heads, and Sensei called out, "Fight!"

I reached out to tap gloves, but my opponent swung at my head instead. He missed. "Ok," I said to myself, "be that way."

I jabbed at his face, hitting him with my left. He swung wildly, missing again. He followed with another punch, which connected by my right ear, but not very hard. I threw a roundhouse kick with my right leg, and the top of my foot connected with the left side of his head. He screamed and his face got red. He came at me swinging violently, but he got nothing but air.

He backed up and I moved forward and delivered a spinning hook kick. He lifted his hands up to block his face, but I had aimed just under his armpit. The spinning hook kick was my most powerful strike. When my heel connected with his ribs, I felt something give and crack.

He collapsed to the mat in a heap and moaned for a moment. Then he ripped off his gloves and threw them at me, running out the door yelling. The Sensei turned around and sauntered into his office without saying a word. The fight had only lasted about one minute. I stood there in the middle of the dojo, my gloves still on, wondering what had just happened.

After my workout, I went into the Sensis's office and asked if the guy I hit was all right. "He's fine," he told me. Then he abruptly changed the topic.

"We have a kickboxing match next month at the Sports Center Ring in Rochester. Would you be ready by then?"

I couldn't say no to Sensei, so I answered, "Yes, I will be ready." So I had my first full-contact kickboxing bout scheduled for the next month. What had I gotten myself into? I had watched a few fights before, and the guys beat each other up pretty badly. At the time, my Sensei was ranked seventh in the world in the PKA (Professional Kickboxing Association). That was pre-MMA or UFC. My fight, however, would be at the amateur level.

On my next work day, I got a call at about 0600 to report to Station One. At 0730, I was already settled in, a cup of joe in my hand. I was talking to the boys from the OFU about the condo fire we had fought three days ago. It was in the newspapers that we had lost five out of ten units in the complex. Not good press for the fire department.

The truth was that we had done a good job stopping the fire at five and not losing the whole thing. While I was on my Kelly days, the fire inspector determined that the fire had started in front of the main entrance of the condos. There had been a large planter with dry, dead plants in it. People would throw paper, garbage and cigarettes in there before going inside. A lit cigarette had been tossed into it, starting the fire. Then the wood siding caught on fire, from which it spread to the attic and roof.

The fire spread so rapidly because there were no fire stops in the attics. When attached condos are built, they are supposed to have a plasterboard wall between the attics of each condo unit. To save a little money, the builder didn't put fire stops in, which was against code. We could have lost men at that fire, especially the ones on the roof.

As we talked, the others from my unit came strolling in. While most everyone gets there early, a few would come in seconds before 0800. We called them "wire men." The wire man from today's shift still wasn't there at

0800. We always tried to have each other's backs, so Wayne, from the other unit, offered to fill in for him.

"Ok, Wayne," Lieutenant accepted. "I had better give Bill a call."

The problem with being a wire man is, of course, you might get held up and be late. Everyone knew they should be there by 0730, and that if they weren't, someone would call them at home. Depending on who was in charge that day, you might get written up for being late. It could vary based on how late you were. The man in charge had the option of writing you up or letting someone work for you. Bill was only five minutes late that time.

Once, we had another wire man who didn't show up on time. We waited a half hour before calling him at home. It turned out that he had slept through his alarm. If we overslept, most of us would throw on our clothes and hurry to the station. Not this guy. He strolled in an hour and a half late. When he was asked why, he said, "I had to take a shower and eat breakfast." I thought for sure he would be written up, but they let it go. He was one of the chosen ones, I guess.

Anyway, we were discussing how one of the Engines had gotten into an accident at the condo fire. The driver had backed into a parked car while trying to reach a hydrant. We were joking with him, asking "Did you write your 'Dear Chief' letter?"

"Yes," he replied. "It said 'Dear Chief, I'm so sorry for breaking your ! @#$% truck." Everyone laughed.

In reality, it was a serous thing to have an accident in a department vehicle. Even though he joked, he was embarrassed and would actually have to write a 'Dear Chief' letter giving his official explanation and apology. It would end up in his personnel file forever.

"Johnson," Lieutenant said, "Did you ever have to write a 'Dear Chief' letter?"

"I have one on file," I said vaguely.

"Ok, tell us."

"A long time ago, far, far away at Station One," I began, "a subby named Johnson, yours truly, was asked by Chief Benson to take the brand new squad to the town hall and fill it with gas." They were all listening to my story intently, no doubt expecting it to be entertaining at the least.

"I remember that the Chief opened the apparatus room door for me, and I got in the vehicle. It had a new car smell. All the new switches and radios on the dash board twinkled in the light. 'This is nice,' I thought to myself as I buckled my seat belt. When I started the engine, I looked at the fuel gauge. It read a hair above E. I put the truck in drive and started my mission.

"Our gas pumps at the station were not working, so I had to use the ones designated for the police, at the old town hall on Orchard Lake Road. The police department was located there also. It was an old brick building, and the patrol cars were kept in back, next to the entrance. There was a canopy between the parking lot and the town hall. I had to drive under the canopy to get to the pumps, so I slowly cruised under it. When I was about halfway through, I heard a thump. I immediately stopped and thought, 'Was that me? Probably not, but
I had better check it out.'

"I got out of the squad and went around back. To my horror, there were two large red round plastic lenses and their chrome base lying on the pavement. I looked up at the rear top of the squad and saw the holes and turned up metal where the lights had been yanked out. My heart sank. I stood for a minute looking at the disaster I had caused.

"'Don't worry,' said a voice at my side. I looked up and saw a woman and a child. 'Don't worry,' she repeated. 'It didn't hurt us.'

"I remember thinking to myself, 'I wasn't worried about you! I just wrecked the brand new squad that hasn't even been on a run yet.'

"I still had to fill the squad gas tank. So I took the big red lights off the pavement and carefully placed them in the back on the stretcher. I carefully maneuvered to the pumps, a large knot in my stomach. I could hardly concentrate on the task of filling the gas tank. The enormity of what I had done was starting to sink in. I was still a subby. Would I get fired? I felt so glum. I wondered what the other firefighters would think. I finished filling the gas tank, then drove the squad, without further incident, back to the station. I backed into the stall and closed the door. 'What will I tell the Chief?' I wondered."

"The Chief met me in the apparatus room. He asked me, 'How did it go?'

"I paused for a moment and replied, 'Not too well, Chief.' 'What do you mean?' he asked."

"I pointed to the back of the squad. When the Chief saw the damage, he dropped his head and shook it. He turned back to the door and said, as he left the apparatus room, 'You know you will have to write a letter.' Then he disappeared behind the door."

One of the guys asked, "What happened to you?"

"I wrote the letter. That's all," I commented. "Although, I wasn't allowed to drive the squad for quite a while."

Just then, Bill ambled through the door. It was 0807. "Thanks for working in for me, Wayne," Bill said. As he got up to leave, Wayne nodded, "Any time."

Bill went into the kitchen to get a cup of coffee, while I proceeded into the apparatus room to check my truck. I was scheduled to drive the Ladder truck. I used to drive it frequently when I was assigned to Station One. This vehicle was fairly new.

The Ladder we had before this one was just as big, but it didn't have a bucket in front. It was also difficult to drive, because it had a manual transmission. The clutch was difficult to push down, so when I had to stop at a long red light, my leg would get rubbery. And that was when I was in great shape! The new Ladder was a lot easier to drive with the automatic transmission.

I gazed at the huge red truck taking up the front and rear bays. The Engine only occupied one bay, but this beast ate up two. A big white ladder was sitting atop the mighty red machine. It was calling to me.

"Start me up. Raise my ladder," she purred.

"Oh baby, I will shortly," I crooned back, "But first I have to check you out."

I went around the front and looked up at the big white bucket that was about five inches away from the door. The nice thing about Station One's apparatus room was that all the doors were lined with windows. It was like being in a glass house with lots of natural light.

As I was checking a side compartment, I saw movement out of the corner of my eye. I turned to look out the door and saw a tire bouncing down the road. Just a tire. It would bounce, then roll then leap up, getting closer and closer. It struck something in the road, skipped up to the sidewalk and kept rolling. This thing was going fast! It was going to roll onto the sidewalk in front of the station. Then the tire veered on a bounce and headed right for our door.

It slammed into the last bay with a loud crash, the impact bending the metal door frame. The glass shattered and blew into the bay. The tire was now wedged into the mangled door. As the chaos came to a stop, I expected everyone to come running, but I was still the only one in the apparatus room.

I walked over to the tire caught in the door, looking out the other bay door to see where it had come from. There was the normal traffic driving by. I had to report the incident, so I went into the living room where everyone was and announced, "A tire just crashed through the apparatus door."

The men looked up for a moment, then went back to what they were doing. I just realized how stupid I sounded. A tire through the bay door. Right. The Lieutenant strolled out of the Chief's office and I called to him.

"Lieutenant, a tire just crashed into the apparatus room door!" I said.

"How come I didn't hear anything?" he asked me.

"I don't know, because it was loud."

"Alright, show me." I led the lieutenant into the apparatus room, the other men following behind. I showed them the damage.

"Well, I'll be @#$% #," cussed the lieutenant. Just then a young man and woman came up to the door.

"The tire came off my truck while we were driving," the man told us. "Our car is about a mile down the road. Can anyone give us a ride home?"

I left the lieutenant to deal with the matter and finished checking out my truck. I checked all the outside compartments to make sure all the equipment was there and in working order. Each compartment had a list of the equipment stored in there. We had chain saws, ring saws, extra air bottles and climbing belts to attach us to the ladder when we climbed up or rode in the bucket. The full list of equipment was quite lengthy. It took a long time to go through the whole truck.

Then I started the engine and pulled it out onto the apron. The Ladder weighed about seventeen thousand pounds, so it took a lot of power to start and stop the monster. After I made sure the fuel tank was full and had checked everything in the cab, I flipped the ladder p.t.o. switch, located between the two front seats.

I could hear it engage. The controls were on the back top of the truck. I walked around to the rear, and saw five levers sticking out of the back. One lever raised and lowered the ladder, and another lever extended and retracted its one-hundred foot length. The next lever rotated the ladder to the right or left.

Before I could move the ladder, I had to lower the outriggers. In the back compartment on each side of the truck was a metal plate measuring about one square foot, which had to be placed on the ground beside the outriggers. One went on each side of the truck. The metal plate had to be the right distance from the truck, or the outrigger would miss it. I measured the distance by using the metal plate as a guide. Two plate lengths away from the outrigger, I set it down on the pavement.

If we failed to put down the outriggers when we extended or turned the ladder, it could, and probably would, tip over the entire truck. I measured and set the other plate on the pavement. At the back, was a switch panel to engage the outriggers. The lever to the far right lowered and raised the right outrigger and the one to the far left controlled the left one. I pulled the left lever down and with a loud whining sound, the outrigger slowly lowered and stopped just above the metal plate. I did the same to the right.

I went to the make sure that the plates were in the perfect position before I put the full weight of the outriggers on them. If necessary, I would slide the plates into a better position.

I went back behind the truck and finished lowering the outriggers. The ladder had a governor so that when I raised or turned the ladder, the truck's engine would rev up to provide the necessary power. While I was turning the ladder, the lieutenant decided to have training.

"Raise and extend the ladder when they get into the bucket," lieutenant called to me. I waited for the three firefighters to don their safety belts and climb into the bucket.

"Ok, raise the ladder," lieutenant commanded. I pushed up on the extending and raising levers at the same time, in order to avoid damaging the ladder. In addition, if I extended the ladder too much to the side, that could also cause damage or even tip the truck over. The ladder was very tough and could take a lot of stress, but even this rig had its limits.

The engine accelerated when I pushed the levers, lifting the bucket and its occupants up into the sky. Eventually, they rose up to about one-hundred feet off the ground. I rotated the ladder to the right, then to the left. The cars on Orchard Lake Road were slowing down, some even stopping on the side of the road to watch. There was a parking lot on the property next to the station where cars pulled in to gawk.

It was pretty exciting to be in control of such an extremely powerful machine. As I maneuvered the ladder, I glanced up between the rungs to the bucket and saw the small men securely enjoying their elevated view.
"Are you ready to go up?" the lieutenant asked me, grinning. "Sure," I replied readily, "I would like to go up."

I slowly retracted and lowered the ladder until it rested on the top of the truck. I handed the controls over to Bill, while I put the safety belt around my waist. Dangling from the yellow safety belt was a carabiner that I would attach to the bucket. I climbed into the bucket along with two other firefighters and clipped onto the inside safety bar.

The engine of the ladder truck revved up and the bucket, with me and the others inside, started to rise. First the bucket jerked, but the ride got smoother as we climbed. We slowly rose almost straight up. Higher and higher we reached. The men on the ground were getting smaller. When the ladder was fully extended, we stopped.

I looked to my right and saw the now small cars driving down Orchard Lake Road. I could even see the town hall from up here. Being up in the ladder's bucket was like a carnival ride. And, like a carnival ride, it was over way too soon.

The ladder started to move with a bounce, beginning the trip back down. The ground edged closer. The bucket was brought smoothly to rest on top of the truck's landing area. Once the bucket slid gently back into place, we released our carabiners and exited.

I had to make sure the ladder was latched down properly so it wouldn't move in transit. Everyone went back inside, while I backed Ladder One into its bay. The lieutenant spotted for me, guiding me safely in. I engaged the parking brake, shut the engine off and went back inside for my next cup of coffee.

This impromptu training session would be recorded, counting toward the hours of drill or training we were required to participate in. The more the better was our general feeling.

"Hey, Johnson," the Captain called to me, as he exited the Chief's office, "I heard you will be fighting next month."

"Yeah. I was asked to be in one of three kickboxing matches before a karate demonstration," I explained. "My Sensei's Sensei will break a boulder with his bare hands after my fight. You're welcome to come and watch."

"I don't think so, but thanks for the invite," the Captain replied, shaking his head.

Then I pointed out something to entice him. "There is a bar in the arena."

"Twist my arm! I'll be there!" Captain said, grinning, as he went back into the office. Just then the tones went off.

"Rescue One, you have a possible heart attack at the JCC (Jewish Community Center) on Maple. Station Two is out on a PIA. Time out, 1034."

"Johnson, you are in the back of the Rescue. Jack is out shopping," the lieutenant said. Normally I wouldn't go on a medical when I am assigned to the Ladder, but of course this wasn't normal. Heck, it never was.

I hopped into the back of the Rescue while Bill drove. Marty rode shot gun. We made a left onto Orchard Lake Road and headed to Maple. We turned right and sped along for about three miles. The JCC was on the right. Technically, it was in Station Two's area, but they were out on a run, so we had to go.

As we approached, I heard Ruth's voice on Engine Two's radio. "Engine Two back in service and responding to the JCC." Ruth was another of our firewomen.

"Rescue One on scene," Marty called in the mic.

"Engine Two on scene," I heard as I hopped out of the back. Bill and Marty helped me with the equipment, and we quickly entered the large building. The JCC had just about everything; a gym, a basketball court, a swimming pool, a squash court and handball courts. There were large locker rooms for men and women. A dark-haired woman met us at the entrance.

She said, "A man is having a heart attack in the men's locker room!" We followed her to the locker room and hurried in.

It was a huge space, filled with a good number of lockers and showers. What was unusual was that it also had a lounge area, where the men could kick back, watch TV or just relax in recliner chairs. The odd thing was that the men lounged in the locker room nude.

We warned them as we entered that we had a woman with us. We were led by another worker through the lounge to the main locker room. There were several nude men resting. I spotted an elderly gentleman lying on the locker room floor between two benches.

Another man, dressed in a pair of underwear, was trying to help, accompanied by another man, who wore nothing at all. That man left as he saw us. Kneeling next to the patient, Ruth asked, "Are you having any chest pain?"

"Yes," came the labored reply. "I have pain in my chest going down my left arm and up into my jaw."

I immediately thought to myself, "You don't get more classic symptoms for an MI (myocardial infarction or heart attack) than that!"

Ruth asked the man about his medical history, medications, etc. The patient felt cool and clammy.

I asked, "What were you doing when the chest pains started?"

"I had just finished playing racquetball, so I was taking a shower. Then the chest pains started," the man answered. "It feels like an elephant is sitting on my chest." I started an IV and Bill gave him oxygen. Marty hooked the patient up to the LIFEPAK monitor.

One guy came into the locker room from the lounge to give us his account of what had caused the heart attack. He stood behind Ruth and bent over to see what was going on. Since he was nude as he hovered over top of Ruth, he was dangling his junk in front of her face. "Get that out of my face, or I will cut it off with a scalpel!" Ruth snapped. The man quickly left, looking sheepish. That story became a favorite of Ruth's to tell.

Meanwhile, the cardiac monitor showed a Q-wave and a raised ST segment. This meant that the heart was not getting enough oxygenated blood and there was cardiac damage. He was indeed having a serious heart attack. He was also throwing PVCs, which meant the cardiac tissue had become irritated because of the accruing injury. A PVC is when the heart prematurely beats backwards. When that happens, the patient can go into cardiac arrest.

I pushed an amp of lidocaine into the IV and the PVCs stopped. Lidocaine worked well for calming cardiac tissue. The patient was in a lot of pain and had trouble breathing. His blood pressure was good, so we gave him Nitroglycerin and morphine. He immediately relaxed. The chest pain quickly went away.

By that time the ambulance crew showed up with the stretcher. We stepped aside to let their crew do the lifting. One of the attendants asked the patient, "Can you walk to the stretcher?"

"I think so," the patient answered.

I said to them, "No! Don't let him walk! Carry him."

"Oh, he can walk," the attendant protested, helping the patient to his feet before I could stop him. The man immediately went into cardiac arrest. Ventricular fibrillation was on the monitor.

"Get him down!" I yelled. The attendant laid the patient back down, looking shocked. "That's why we don't let cardiac patients get up!" I snapped.

"Charging paddles to 200!" Marty called out. The LIFEPAK whined as the paddles charged. Placing the paddles on the patient's chest, Marty yelled, "Clear!"

He discharged the paddles and the patient jumped, but there was no change. "Charging to 360 Jules!" Marty called, setting the paddles on the man's chest. "Clear!" He pushed the buttons on the paddles. With a thump, the patient lurched. We waited for a few seconds. The ECG showed normal sinus rhythm.

"Checking pulse," I said, placing my fingers against the artery in his neck. "I have a pulse." After a moment, I added, "And the patient is breathing, but he's still unconscious. Let's get him packed up. This time carry him!"

The patient was loaded onto the stretcher and brought out to the ambulance. He regained consciousness on the way to the hospital. Fortunately for him, the guy ended up walking out of the hospital a few days later. Sadly, that is pretty unusual.

It seems that we have had more success with older people in cardiac arrest then with younger patients. In part that's because older people have collateral circulation. When an older heart has partial obstruction of the cardiac arteries, it develops extra arteries. Younger hearts have wide-open, large arteries with no collateral circulation.
As a result, they usually do not do well because blood clots will kill a large amount of cardiac muscle.

When we got back to the station, we talked about that run while Jack was fixing lunch. "It is not too often when we get a save," Marty pointed out.

"No. It's nice for a change," I agreed. It's not like TV where everyone in cardiac arrest comes back. On the rare occasions when they do, rarely do they walk out of the hospital. It depends on what caused the cardiac arrest and how long the person was in arrest. If the person has a blood clot in a main artery, too much of the heart is affected and the patient probably won't make it.

If cardiac arrest was caused by electrocution and defibrillation is done quickly, the patient has a good chance. The same is true with drowning. Speed is the key. The only way to convert someone in ventricular fibrillation is electric defibrillation. That's why automatic defibrillators or AED stations are so important.

"How about Ruth taking on the guy who was dangling his junk?" Bill said.

"Yeah!" I said. "She sent him away with his tail between his legs." We all laughed.

"She would have done it too," Bill added.

"Done what?" asked Jack from the kitchen.

"Cut his junk off with a scalpel."

"She said that?" Jack asked, his eyes wide with disbelief.

"Yes she did," I answered, nodding my head.

Jack started setting the table for lunch. We were having hotdogs and hamburgers, chips and dip. We helped get the table ready. After Jack called everyone to eat, we crowded around the lunch table. Even the Captain and Chief joined us. The mood was fairly jolly as we prepared to enjoy our meal.

Until the tones went off.

# Chapter 23 - Sometimes You Kick, Sometimes You Get Kicked

"Station Three you have an automatic alarm at 3200 Green Lake Road."

"That place again?" I commented. I recognized the address as one we had been to multiple times for false alarms. Fortunately, it was Station Three's run this time. We at Station One could enjoy our lunch without interruption. Chances were, it would be a false alarm. Something other than fire always seemed to set those automatic alarms off, so we were in the habit of only sending one Engine. But we still had to be ready, because one in ten could be an actual fire.

After lunch, the Chief stepped out of his office and called for me, "Johnson! In my office."

"Now what did I do?" I thought miserably to myself. I opened the office door and walked in.

"Yes, Chief?" "I need you back at Station Three," the Chief told me. "Do you want to go back there?"

"Yes, Chief! I would like that," I replied, nodding.

"Good. You are transferred to Three starting next month," he announced.

"Great!" I smiled.

As I started to walk out, the Chief said, "Wait, Johnson! One more thing." I stopped and turned back to listen. "You are being promoted to Sergeant. There will be a ceremony next month for the men receiving promotions."

"Thank you, Chief," I said, feeling pleasantly surprised.

The Chief shook his head, saying, "I don't understand why people want to be stationed at the outhouses."

He always called Stations Three and Four "the outhouses."

"Now get out of here so I can finish my paperwork." I was going home to Station Three. I practically skipped out of the office. Nothing could ruin my mood now, except…I heard the tones go off, followed by "Station One. Respond to a man with chest pains at 2435 Walnut Lake Road. Time out, 1530."

I met Bill and Marty at the Rescue. We climbed in and took off.

"Rescue One enroute to 2435 Walnut Lake Road," Marty called in as we turned left onto Orchard Lake Road.

"Enroute received, Rescue One." When we arrived at the house, I jumped out with the equipment. Marty and Bill met me and helped carried the gear to the house. As I knocked on the door, a little snow started to fall. A lady in her mid-thirties soon came to the door. "He's in here." She led us to the living room. A man in his early forties was lying on a couch.

He said with an apologetic smile, "Hi guys. I'm sorry to bother you. I'm sure it's nothing. My name is Jeff."

"No bother," I assured him, "this is what we get paid for."

Marty said, "What's bothering you?"

"I have a little tickle in my chest," Jeff replied, "but I feel fine. My wife called. I told her not to."

"Well, let us check you out and we'll get out of your hair," I assured him.

"Ok, ok," he agreed, "but I'm fine." Their two children were playing in the dining room nearby. They were about ten and eleven years old.

"Let me check your blood pressure," I said, picking up the blood pressure cuff. I wrapped it around his arm and then his eyes rolled back into his head. He started seizing. His whole body shook violently. He was in what looked like a grand mal seizure, but it wasn't. We could tell that he had gone into cardiac arrest right in front of us. All of us were stunned for a moment.

The guy had been just fine a moment ago. I went to check his pulse. He made gasping noises as his body tried to breathe. "He doesn't have a pulse!" I yelled.

Marty got out the paddles and handed them to me. "I'll start the IV," he said. The seizures slowed, and Bill took the stethoscope to listen to his chest. "No heart beat!" he told us.

The patient's wife was standing behind us yelling, "What's happening? What's happening?"

"Let's get him on the floor," I said. The three of us lifted him to the floor. The children came to see what was going on. I put the gel pads on his chest and set the paddles there to see the heart rhythm.

"V-fib," I announced, charging the paddles to 200 Jules. I placed the paddles on the gel pads, and yelled, "Clear!" while depressing the two red buttons at the same time. Thump! The electric charge was released through the patient's chest. His body jumped. The seizures had stopped, but when I looked at the monitor, I could see he was still in V-fib.

"No change" I yelled, "charging to 300 Jules!" All of a sudden, I felt the patient's body moving. I looked down at his feet and saw two yellow hound dogs, one attached to each leg, violently humping and howling. Obviously upset with what was happening to their master, the dogs had become excited and did what dogs do. They didn't realize why they were feeling this way.

Stunned by the dogs' behavior for a moment, I yelled, "Someone get these dogs out of here!" The wife and kids grabbed the dogs off their master and put them into a room. Then we went back to work. I charged the paddles again, slapped them on his chest and yelled, "Clear!" His body jumped, then I waited for the ECG to steady.

"Still in V-fib," I said again. "Charging to 360 Jules! Clear!" I pushed the red buttons. The patient's body jerked again and I looked at the monitor, waiting for it to settle down.

"Still in V-fib!" I said. "Start CPR!"

Bill started compressions and Marty started an IV. I worked on his airway. I got the tube in right away and started ventilating him with a bag mask. Marty got the IV in and gave him epinephrine IVP.

"Try again!" Marty called out. I charged the defibrillator again.

After the charging whine stopped, I yelled, "Clear!"

I put the paddles to his chest and pushed the buttons. The patient jumped as the electricity ran through his body. We waited for the monitor to steady. "Still in V-fib!" I shouted.

"Try lidocaine!" Marty called out. I was already picking up the vial. I pushed in the proper amount of lidocaine as CPR continued.

"Charging again," I said. When it was ready, I yelled "Clear!" and defibrillated again. The monitor read.... V-fib. By that time the ambulance crew arrived with their stretcher. The police had also arrived and had taken the family into a back room while we worked.

"Let's pack him up and get going," I said in frustration. We all knew that there wasn't much chance of bringing him back now, but we would keep trying.

We loaded him into the back of the ambulance and started on our way. Marty and I and one of the ambulance attendees were in back with the patient. Just before we left, I tried atropine. At that time, it was a new drug used to treat cardiac arrest. It speeds up a slow heart rate. It was found to have some success in V-fib patients. I pushed in the atropine and charged the paddles again. "Clear!" I barked, putting the paddles to his chest. I released the shock and the body lurched.

"V-fib still," I said, charging the paddles again. I defibrillated him several more times with no success. We gave him most every drug that we had in the box, but nothing worked. Inter-cardiac injections were no longer an approved treatment, so there wasn't much more we could do. When we arrived at the hospital, the patient was quickly taken to a cardiac care room. There the doctors and nurses worked on him for over an hour.

A couple of times they were able to get a ventricular rhythm for a short time, but eventually he went flat line and they called it. We were told good work by the head doctor, but that didn't make us feel much better.

I kept picturing his kids, standing next to their terrified mother. I helped Marty do the paperwork and restock the drug box at the pharmacy.

"Let's get out of here!" he said when we were finally finished. We talked about the run on the way back. "We did everything that we could do. It just was his time."

Normally it doesn't bother me about losing a patient when they are fairly old and have lived their lives. But this guy had a wife and young children and had been in good health. Worst of all, he died in front of his family.

The night of my scheduled fight arrived. I had been working out every day at the dojo, as well as the stations and at home. I worked out three hours a day.

During the fight day I didn't do much. I just watched TV and lounged. There were going to be several guys from the department there to see me get my block knocked off. All the same, I was as ready as I could be.

People were gathering at the Sports Center Ring. I had never been there before. I saw some of the men I worked with when I arrived, but I was focused on getting prepped.

I wore a white gi bottom, with no top. I had my hands wrapped with cotton strips and tape. I got my gloves on and the Sensei put Vaseline on my face to help prevent cuts.

I had to sit and watch some karate demonstrations and two fights before it would be my turn. Then some board and brick breaking took place. Then they had to clean up the ring to get it ready for the match. The ring looked like a regular boxing ring, except that it backed up to a wall and the crowd was in front and on the sides.

When it was time, the announcer called my name and my opponent's name. We entered the ring and I looked at the crowd. I saw it was full. I caught a glimpse of the Captain, a drink in his hand, talking to some blond. I spotted my wife next to her friend.

The bell rang and the referee called us to the center. He gave us the usual. No hitting below the belt, no biting, and so on. I looked at my opponent. He looked familiar. I thought I'd seen him around the dojo. We sized each other up, me at five feet seven and him at six feet two. His head was going to be hard to reach.

"Touch gloves and fight!" the referee shouted.

We touched gloves, and it started. I attacked first, throwing a roundhouse kick to his abdomen. It made contact and my opponent groaned and backed up. He came at me, throwing punches.

It all seemed to happen in slow motion. One punch was aimed straight at my nose. I ducked, and he missed. Another punch from his right was coming over my left shoulder. I was able to evade that one. A third punch came over my right shoulder and I easily dodged that.

He was now wide open. I reacted with a full-force punch between his gloves, slamming into his jaw. He went down to the floor, but he got back up. The referee sent me to my corner. My opponent was given a standing eight count. The ref asked him "Are you able to continue?" He shook his head yes.

"Fight!" the ref said again. When we were close enough, I jabbed, but missed. He tried a front kick and hit my elbow. I threw a spinning hook kick. I thought I had him, but he backed up just in time, and I missed. He came at me, punching, and I evaded him.

Again, he was open for a split second and between his gloves was his jaw. My right fist hit the target and he fell to the floor. My opponent got back up, and the bell rang. We had a two minute break between each round. We still had two more rounds, and I was worn out. My legs felt rubbery.

Sensei said, "You have to go three rounds to allow my Sensei to get ready for his boulder breaking." I nodded, unsure I could last that long, but determined to try. The bell rang and the referee called us to the center again and said, "Fight!"

We touched gloves again, and my opponent punched first, connecting with my shoulder. I didn't feel anything. I threw a front kick, which he blocked. I threw a side kick, which fell short. However I followed up with a right that connected to his jaw. Down he went. I went to my corner while he got a standing eight count.

During the eight count, my Sensei reminded me, "Stretch the fight out so we can get ready."

I thought, "How can I do that? He's trying to knock me out!"

"Fight!" The referee shouted again. I suddenly got my second wind. I felt strong. I started out with a round house kick, hitting him in the abdomen. He bent over and groaned, which made his jaw a big target. And I did not miss. He fell to the floor again.

I thought, "Call it. Stop the fight. He has had enough." Sure enough, the referee stopped the contest. He took my arm and raised it into the air. I looked over to my opponent, who was on his feet. I went over to him and put my arm around him and said, "Good fight."

He looked at me but didn't respond. "Are you all right?" I asked. He nodded his head yes and said, "Good fight." I patted him on the back and went into the locker room. There was no shower, so I slid on my clothes and went out to see the rest of the show. When I reached my wife she said, "Good job."

Then a young man, about my size, said to me, "Come on over to the bar and let me buy you a drink. It's good to see someone our size deck a big guy."

"Thanks," I said, adding, "I'll have a Coke."

After the show was over and everyone had left, Sensei asked me if I could give someone a lift back to the dojo. Of course I agreed; I couldn't say no to Sensei.

"Tom needs a ride," Sensei said, indicating the man walking out. It was the guy I had just knocked out. It was an awkward ride back.

The next day I was at Station One. The Captain found me and said, "Great fight. I had a good time last night."

"Thanks, I saw you. You were with a blond, right?" I commented. The Captain smiled mysteriously, chuckled, then turned and disappeared into his office with his coffee.

Everyone treated me differently for a while after my fight, like they had a new respect for me. I paid a price for the glory, though. I sure was in pain that day.

"I shouldn't be sore," I thought. "He didn't lay a glove on me that I remember." My foot was sore, my hands were sore, my knee was sore and I had a bruise under my left eye. How was it that I easily won my fight and yet I was still beat up?

I had a hard time getting things done at work that day. I decided I would retire from fighting. The Fire Department was more important than winning mixed martial arts fights. If I got hurt, I could lose my job. Besides, I had done enough to cross it off my bucket list.

# Chapter 24 - Winter Wonderland

It was November, and I was assigned to Station Three once again. It was starting to get cold and even to snow a little. I was sitting at the kitchen table with Bob when he asked me, "When are you going deer hunting this year?"

"Oh, I can't go this year, at least not on opening day. I'm scheduled to work," I replied. My work day fell right on November 15th that year and no one would trade that day out with me. Believe me, I tried everyone possible. "I may go up north at the end of the month," I added. It was snowing harder as we talked.

"I think it will be an early winter this year," Bob predicted, staring at the falling snow. Little did we know that snow would be our adversary that evening. Nothing much happened during the day, except for a smoke investigation. I had just returned from grocery shopping when the run had come in.

"Station three," Dispatch called, "you have a smoke investigation at 6577 Green Lake Road. Woman smells smoke in her house. Time out, 0930."

We took the map and I pulled the Engine right onto Green Lake Road. "Engine Three enroute to 6577 Green Lake Road."

"Enroute received, Engine Three. Be advised a patrol car is on the way." The address was only down the street, and we arrived in less than a minute.

"Engine Three on scene, along with police, nothing visible," we called in.

The police car had arrived at about the same time as us. Bob, Officer Miller and I walked up to the beautiful house on Green Lake. Bob rang the doorbell, and a young woman answered it. She calmly greeted us, saying, "Hi boys! Come in. This way."

My eyes were not used to the dark house, so I couldn't really see what we were getting in to. She led us down a hallway to the laundry room. Turning on the lights, she told us, "I smelled it in here."

"What did you smell?" I asked. My eyes were starting to get used to the low light.

"I smelled something when I turned on the dryer," she answered. My eyes were now adjusted. She was a slender young woman wearing a tight, almost see-through long black nightgown. Being professional, I wouldn't notice a thing like that, but she stuck out like a…well let's just say she stuck out. The sheer nightgown clung to her body and hid nothing.

"Bob," I said. No response. "Bob!" I repeated, a little more forcefully. "Bob. Bob!"

He finally looked, startled from his trance, and said, "What?" Then he came more to his senses and asked her, "Oh, Ma'am can you start the dryer?" He smiled at her.

"Sure. Just a minute," she said, bending over to pull the clothes out first. This motion revealed her large breasts, and she acted like she didn't notice. Then she reached over and turned on the dryer. It ran for a while, but we didn't smell anything. I tried to keep my eyes averted, but it wasn't easy. In fact, I'll admit I failed.

"I don't smell anything unusual, Ma'am," Bob stated.

"Well, I'm sure I smelled something," she replied. "Oh, wait. It was down in the basement. This way."

She waved for us to follow. I tried not to notice that the nightgown clung to her curves and showed her backside in great detail, bouncing with every step. When she flipped on the light switch, we saw that it was a finished basement, complete with a pool table and a couch with a bed pulled out. Folded sheets lay on top of it. No one said anything. I finally broke the awkward silence.

"What did you smell, exactly? Where did you smell it?"

"I smelled it right in here."

"I don't smelling anything," I said.

"I might smell something," Officer Miller said.

Bob asked, "Did you turn on the furnace this morning?"

"Yes, yes! That must be it," she said in an innocent voice. We spent some amount of time standing there.

Finally, Bob said, "Well, whatever it was, it's gone now."

"I know I smelled something," she insisted.

"We have to get back in service," Bob explained. "Feel free to call if you smell it again."

"Ok, I will," she said as she walked towards the door to the upstairs. She turned back to us and waved as her chest bounced back and forth under her gown. "Are you boys coming?" she asked.

We followed her back up the stairs and down the hallway to the front door. "I don't understand what happened," she said, apologetically. "Everything was fine until my husband left this morning. He leaves for work every morning at exactly 8:30 and doesn't get home until 8:00 at night."

We walked out the door and I said, "Call us if you need us."

"Thank you," she said as she closed the door.

Officer Miller came up to Bob and me. He asked, "So, do you think she was trolling?"

Bob and I said at the same time, "Nooo!" Then I pointed out, "I guess she could have put on a robe, but that wouldn't have attracted as much attention."

"I think she was getting cold," Bob said. Like a dummy I asked,

"How do you know…ooh, never mind," I added, as I figured it out.

Then Officer Miller said, "I think she was lonely."

She never called again that I know of, but rumor had it that Officer Miller may have visited her the next morning, just to see if she was alright. That was the highlight of the day. But that night was a different story.

Tones went off as I was lifting weights in the bunk room. "Station Four, Station Three, respond to a snowmobile accident at 3000 Parkway in Zox sub. Time out, 2008."

The first day of snow and already there was an accident.

"Engine Four, Rescue Four responding," the Lieutenant of Station Four called in.

"Engine Three responding," Bob called into the mic.

"Engine Four, Rescue Four, Engine Three responding," repeated the dispatcher.

"Be advised we have gotten several calls saying snowmobile verses car on the bridge."

It wasn't far from Station Four to the bridge in question.

"Engine Four, Rescue Four on scene," we heard just before we arrived.

"On scene received," Dispatch responded.

A minute later we heard, "Engine Four reporting two snowmobiles and a car involved with mutable injuries."

We didn't have to say anything to each other because we have had serious car accidents at that location before. We pulled up to the small bridge that ran over a narrow canal. In Zox subdivision, there are a series of canals with houses alongside them. A road that connects the sub together is linked by a series of arched bridges that are not known for great visibility of oncoming traffic.

It was dark out now and the red and blue lights of the police and fire vehicles reflected off the white snow. Engine Four had its spot lights illuminating the scene. There was one snowmobile on the far side of the bridge and one on our side. Two bodies lay a few feet away from the snowmobile nearest us. There was a lot of screaming in the air, coming from injured riders and bystanders.

There were five firefighters on duty at Station Four that day. Three were across the bridge and two were with the injured persons near us. Our Lieutenant, who was directing the scene, said to me.

"G.J. (G.J was yet another of my nicknames), help John with these two." Without replying, I ran up to the mangled bodies.

When I got there John said, "There isn't much we can do for them. They both have brain matter coming out of their fractured skulls."

I looked down at the brightly lit scene. Lying on the snow were two teenagers in a pool of blood. I checked for a pulse, but there was none for either one. It was obvious that with the injuries they had sustained, there was nothing we could do to save them.

One was young, maybe thirteen, lying on his side in the snow. He had a bone sticking out of his upper arm. He also had brain matter coming out of his right temple. I could see the skid marks showing where he had landed on top of the bridge, where he likely hit his head on the steel girder. He must have slid across the roadway to where his body rested now.

The second teen, whom we later discovered was his older brother, was still under the torn up snowmobile. He was lying under the machine on his back with fluid running out of his ears and nose. His one eye was open, but the other eye was missing from the crushed eye socket. Blood and brain matter flowed out of where the eye used to be. He also had no pulse.

It was about thirty degrees out and steam floated up from their bodies. Officer Miller told us, "I've called the ME. They should be here soon."

"Good," said Lieutenant. Officer Miller had learned that three boys, the two brothers and a neighbor, had been jumping the bridge side by side. They didn't see the car coming.

He told us, "Kids like to take their snowmobiles and jump the bridge because it's short and steep. If they go fast enough, they hit the front like a ramp and go airborne, landing on the down side of the bridge." After a pause, he continued, "They did that last year and we had a few complaints. The driver of the car they hit is pretty shaken up. She's sitting in the patrol car with Officer Cooper."

"It wasn't her fault," I commented, knowing that the truth of that wouldn't make it easier for the driver to cope with this experience.

Bob retrieved two blankets out of the Engine and brought them over. I covered the body under the mangled snowmobile, then went over to the other teen and covered his body with the second blanket.

The car that was involved was still on the far side of the bridge. I could see damage on the hood and roof. There was nothing more we could do, so Lieutenant asked me to help with the other patient.

By the time I got over to him, he was already packaged up and ready to be transported. He had an open femur fracture, a fractured elbow and broken clavicle. He was lying on a long back board with a cervical collar on his neck and an IV in his arm.

I helped lift the patient onto the stretcher and into the back of the ambulance. His parents were there consoling him. They were all crying. I shut the ambulance door and it left for the hospital. I walked through the snow back to the other side of the bridge where the two victims lay, the parents crying over their covered bodies.

Neighbors were trying to console them, but I know that nothing can take away the pain they must have felt. The Lieutenant came up to me and asked, "Are you going to do the medical reports on these two?"

"Sure, Lieutenant," I said. "That will be a lot of paper work." I thought to myself. The ME arrived and picked up the bodies. A wrecker came and picked up the torn up snowmobiles. The police were measuring the skid marks and trying to gather the information needed for their investigation.

The Lieutenant told Bob and I that Engine Three could head back.

"Engine Three in service," Bob said, as I backed the Engine onto the road. In my rear view mirror I could still see blue and red lights flashing off the freshly fallen snow. That was the last run of the shift. It took about an hour to finish the medical reports. Then I made my weary way to the bunk room for a few hours respite.

The next time I worked, it was at Station Four. I arrived at 0730 hours, as always, and sat at the kitchen table with the OFU and Lieutenant Bigger. We were sipping our coffee, talking about the snowmobile accident.

The tones interrupted. "Station One, respond to a car hit by a train on Orchard Lake Road and Roosevelt on the train track."

It wasn't for us, so we went back to drinking our coffee. Those tracks have since been pulled up and removed. We ended up discussing the snowmobile accident again.

"Kids are so stupid," Lieutenant Bigger said. "They can't understand the danger of speed and not being able to see where they are going."

"What a waste!" I said. "I can't even begin to imagine what the parents are going through." I paused, before adding, "But, that is why people say 'youth is wasted on the young.'"

Then we moved onto a more lighthearted subject: the lady in the tight nightgown.

After I was done checking the Rescue, Lieutenant Bigger told me that he wanted to ride shotgun with us that day. He must have cursed us, because the tones went off right after he said that.

"Station One, Rescue Four and Engine Two. Respond to Maple and Middle Belt Road for a PIA. An unconscious woman in a car crashed against a tree. Time out, 0905. Be advised Station One and Rescue Two are still out on the car/train accident."

"Well, John," I said to the Lieutenant, "Let's go." It had snowed all through my Kelly and was still snowing very hard now. I felt a bit concerned, because we had been having traction issues lately with the new front tires. This run was so far away in Station One's area, and it was now rush hour.

We left the apparatus room with the lights on and the siren going. As soon as we pulled onto Greer Road and tried to turn left, we went straight instead. I had to slow almost to a stop to finally get the Rescue to turn. Not a good start to the run.

I turned back onto the road and went a little faster, but I had to stop at Hiller and Greer for a red light. I slowly stepped on the brakes and we slid into the intersection, just missing two cars.

"Watch out! Look out for that car!" cried John. It was clear I would have to be a lot more careful than I was used to.

"I can't believe you missed those cars!" John added in disbelief. It was unsettling, the lack of steering control I had. The traffic stopped long enough for us to turn right onto Hiller. When we reached the top of the hill we could see that about a half mile long line of cars lay before us, backed up at the intersection of Hiller and Commerce. Our siren was wailing, and John was repeatedly pushed the air horn. I pulled the Rescue onto the shoulder and attempted to push past the traffic, nearly clipping three cars along the way.

The gravel on the shoulder gave me a little more traction, and I was able to slide the Rescue past the cars. We reached the inter- section, which was at a standstill in all directions. All of the lanes were blocked. I had to stop to wait for a car to get out of the way, but nobody could move. John honked the air horn over and over, with
no effect.

Finally a driver pulled off the road. I attempted to drive through the vacancy. I slid, almost hitting the car next to me. Another car tried to beat us through the opening left by the responsible driver. John lowered the window and stuck his head out to yell at the drivers, "Get out of the way! Get out of the way, idiot!"

Finally, the cars moved. We were able to maneuver through the opening and go straight through the intersection onto Old Orchard Trail. We were making fairly good time on the winding road around the lake. The Rescue slid a lot, but I was able to maintain control until we reached the next intersection.

We were almost to Old Orchard Trail and Pontiac Trail when I heard, "Rescue Four. Be advised that the lady in the car is in cardiac arrest."

"Oh boy," I said as John picked up the mic and responded. "Ok, dispatch, but it will take a while for us to get there due to traffic and conditions."

I slowed to a stop at a red light, and then waited for the traffic to stop. Finally I was able to go. When I stepped on the gas, we went nowhere. We were on the side of a hill and couldn't get enough traction to make it up the incline and through the light. The wheels spun and spun, before grabbing the road surface for a moment and then spinning again.

"John," I said nervously, "I don't think we will make it to the scene." The tires finally grabbed again, and we went through the light. I turned the steering wheel to the left to get onto Pontiac Trail, but we went straight again, almost hitting a car exiting a driveway. We began to slide sideways towards the ditch, but the gravel on the shoulder gave us enough traction to turn back onto the road.

Gravel, mud and slush splashed and crackled under the truck and on the wind shield. I turned on the wipers, and accelerated to about thirty mph until we reached Orchard Lake Road. We were heading for the intersection, and as luck would have it, the light was red. We were traveling downhill this time, toward the light. It became clear that we were not going to be able to stop.

The siren was in Hi/Lo mode, and John was yelling out the window while working the air horn. The intersection was clear for a change, which was a good thing, because we were not going to make the right-hand turn. The back of the Rescue turned, but not the front.

Instead, it slid sideways into the intersection, facing the wrong direction and skated toward the curb. We hit the concrete curb with a bang. The truck tipped to the side on two of its wheels. I found my side lifted up in the air for what seemed like an eternity before we bounced back onto the pavement. I may have hit my head on the ceiling, but I was too shaken to notice until later.

After the truck stopped bobbling, I turned back around and proceeded south onto Orchard Lake Road. Now it was a straight shot to Maple.

"Dispatch to Rescue Four."

"Go ahead, dispatch," we called in.

"Maple is closed. Take Walnut to Middle Belt."

"Message received, dispatch."

"Rescue Four," dispatch came back almost immediately. "I just learned that Walnut Lake Road is closed as well. You will have to take a side street through a subdivision."

"Ok, dispatch," we replied.

To John I said, "We're not going very fast. You have time to find a way through the sub." John picked up the map and quickly found a route. "Turn left here."

I was driving with one tire on the shoulder now, so I was able to make the turn without sliding past. It was a winding, snow-covered subdivision road. When I had to turn, the truck wanted to go straight again. I slowed to a crawl and was able to stay on the road through the S turns.

At one point, the wheels didn't respond when I tried to steer. We were going to crash into a stop sign, and I couldn't even stop. I turned the wheel harder but the truck still went straight. We got closer and closer to the sign. The Rescue veered just a little, somehow missing the sign and getting us through the intersection. We kept going.

It was snowing even more by then, and it was getting harder to see. We came to a T-junction in the road. I pressed the brake lightly, but I could tell we were going to hit the stop sign and plow into a snowy yard.

I took my foot off the brakes, causing the Rescue to lurch to the left, just missing the sign. However, we ran into a yard. All I could think of was that if we got stuck in the snow, we would not make it to the cardiac arrest. The yard we slid into was a snow-covered hill with a clump of evergreen trees halfway up. We plowed into the snow and went up the hill beside the trees.

"Gun it!" John yelled. So I did. We churned through the snow and around the trees. We were near the top of the hill when gravity helped us finish the job. We half slid, half drove around the trees, down the hill and back onto the road. From there we arrived at the accident scene a minute later.

We came to a stop in front of Engine Two and a police car. We were shaking from the crazy ride we'd just had, but we managed to get to the patient. Engine Two's crew and a police officer were performing CPR on the lady, who was now lying on the ground.

"Let's get her into the back of the Rescue," I suggested. We lifted her up into the back. A man stuck his head in the door and said, "I am an ER doctor at St. Thomas' Hospital. Let me help."

We could only let a doctor help if he wanted to take responsibility for the run and would sign a document to that effect. Usually they decline and leave. But this doctor agreed to take charge of the cardiac arrest. He climbed in back with us. I was glad he was there, because John and I were so shaken from the ride here that neither one of us could have started an IV.

He wanted to start a central line, subclavian. A subclavian IV is a long big-bore needle inserted just under the clavicle into the subclavian vein. That is something that we didn't have any training to do.

"Ok," I said, nodding. "I'll get the biggest, longest needle we have." I got out the needle and gave it to him. Then I got an IV bag and tubing, then spiked the IV. The doctor got the subclavian and plugged the IV line into it.

Meanwhile John had put the woman, who looked to be about 50 years old, on the LIFEPAK. The monitor showed a-systole (straight line). We continued CPR. I intubated her and the doctor ordered the drugs, but she never responded. The doctor summed it up, saying, "She picked a bad time to have a heart attack."

When we reached the hospital, it didn't take long for the ER doctors to officially pronounce her dead. By the time we left the hospital, the roads were salted and wet. Not nearly as treacherous as they had been earlier.

The volunteer doctor rode with us back to retrieve his car. On the way, we told the doctor about our hair-raising ride. We also shared our appreciation for his help. After we dropped him off at his car on Middle Belt, we dropped off Jeff, who had driven our Rescue truck to the hospital for us, back to Station Two. It was a slow trip back to Station Four.

We relaxed over a lunch of comfort food: grilled cheese and tomato soup, served with chips and dip.

"I can't believe that we missed all those cars and signs and went up and around the trees barreling through the snow," John said.

"Yes, it was quite a ride," I agreed. "Let's do it again sometime," I added sarcastically.

# Chapter 25 - Their Own Worst Enemy

Sometimes, patients just make things so difficult for us to help them. That can be very frustrating for someone trying to save their life. It was that kind of day.

"Station Four, you have a possible cardiac arrest at the Hiller Road Party Store." We would all have to go on this run, because we only had four men on duty. "Time out, 1511." Hiller Party Store was right across the road from our station.

"Engine Four, Rescue Four responding."

"Engine Four, Rescue Four responding received," Dispatch returned. "The caller says the patient is lying in the doorway."

"Engine Four, Rescue Four on scene," we called almost immediately. As we got out, we saw the patient lying in the middle of the doorway. He was a 70 year-old man, on his back and not moving. We set the equipment next to the patient, and I checked his pulse. I could tell that he was in cardiac arrest just by looking at him. However, we have to check anyway. He had no pulse and was not breathing. I ripped open his shirt to bare his chest, while John got out the LIFEPAK.

"Start CPR," I said. I got out the bag mask and ventilated the patient while Marty did compressions. John was prepping the LIFEPAK. The patient was suddenly trying to get up. He pushed the bag mask away from his face.

"Check pulse," I called out as we stopped CPR. "The man is trying to breathe." He made snoring noises as he struggled to breathe. I checked for a pulse, but couldn't find one.

"I can't feel a pulse," I said. "Marty, see if you can feel it." I hated to second guess myself, but I had never seen someone in arrest try to get up before.

"I can't find a pulse either," Marty said. "Put the paddles on him. He's in V-fib. Continue CPR." Marty started compressions again while John attached the LIFEPAK electrodes to the patient. I tried to bag him, but the patient pushed it away again. We all were second guessing ourselves now. We stopped CPR and checked for a pulse again; there was none.

We looked at the monitor, and it showed V-fib. "John, check the electrodes to make sure that they are in place." Sometimes if an electrode fell off or was loose, it would falsely show V-fib.

"Electrodes have good placement," John reported with a confused look. The patient started to relax.

"Start CPR!" I yelled. We started the compressions and bagging. Once more, he pushed the bag mask away and seemed to try to get up. We stopped again to check his pulse and the monitor. Still no pulse, and leads in the right position.

"Look for a loose wire," I called out. Everything checked out. Then the patient started to relax and we realized that maybe CPR was giving him enough oxygen to move. We just didn't know.

"Continue CPR." It was clear that he was in V-fib.

John gave me the gel patches and I placed them in the proper positions on his chest. He set the paddles on the gel pads. The monitor still read ventricular fibrillation.

"Charging to 200 Jules," John called out. He charged the paddles, which made a whizzzzzzz noise. When it stopped, John positioned the paddles on the gel and yelled, "Clear!"

He released the electricity through the patient's chest, and the body jumped. We waited for the monitor to clear after the defibrillation. I didn't expect much. I was surprised to see NSR, or normal sinus rhythm.

I cried out, "Sinus rhythm! Checking for pulse. I have a pulse!"

"He's breathing!" John started the IV. On the monitor, we could see NSR, with a lot of PVC's. Those are dangerous and can cause the patient to go back into V-fib.

"Let's give him some lidocaine. That should stop the PVC's." I was getting the lidocaine out of the drug box when I heard, "He's in V-fib again! Charging to 200."

I heard the whizzzzzzzzz sound, then John calling "Clear!" The body lurched again.

"We have a rhythm and a pulse," I said. I finally was able to push in the lidocaine.

Bob was now bagging the patient. He said, "He is trying to breathe again."

"Let's get him into the truck," John suggested. We lifted the patient onto our stretcher and put him into the back of our Rescue. John and I were in the back with the patient, and Marty drove. Just after we left the store, he went into cardiac arrest again.

"Patient in V-fib!" I announced. This time John was bagging the patient, so I took the paddles and charged to 200 Jules.

I placed them on his chest and yelled, "Clear!" I pushed the red buttons on the paddles, and the patient jumped. I looked at the monitor and it showed V-fib. "Charging to 300 Jules! Clear!" The patient lurched again.

"He's in a ventricular rhythm." I said, reaching over to feel for a pulse. "I have a pulse."

He may have had a pulse, but he was not breathing. John had to keep ventilating him with the bag mask. We waited for a little bit to see if he would arrest again.

Then I called the hospital. "Rescue Four to St. Thomas' Hospital."

"Go ahead Rescue Four, this is hospital ER."

"We are enroute to your facility with a seventy-year old man that we found in cardiac arrest. It only took us a minute or two to reach him, and we've started CPR and defibrillated four times. We have a line and gave him lidocaine. He has a pulse now, but it is ventricular." I continued filling the ER in. "We don't have his medical history and our ETA is ten minutes."

"Ok, Rescue Four, send us a strip." I transmitted the ECG strip over the radio to the hospital.

"Rescue Four, continue what you are doing and call back if anything changes."

"Ok, Rescue Four out." As I turned off the radio, John called out, "V-fib again!"

I dropped the radio and went for the paddles. "Charging to 360 Jules!" I called out. Once the whizzzzzzzzz stopped, I discharged the paddles. "Clear!" Thump! The monitor was now showing fine fib, which is smaller than regular fib, also known as coarse fib. It does not convert very easily.

"Giving epinephrine," I stated, pushing epinephrine into the IV. "Charging to 360 Jules," I reported. I put the paddles back on his chest and released the shock again.

"Coarse V-fib. Charging to 360. Clear!" Thump! When the monitor cleared it was straight line. "Flat line!" I cried. Flat line means there is no electrical activity in the heart. They don't usually come out of that.

"Ok," I said, feeling desperate, "giving another amp of epinephrine." I pushed it through the IV and started compressions. The patient went to fine fib then to coarse fib.

"Defibbing again!" I charged the paddles to 360 Jules and delivered the shock and waited... and waited. A wide ventricular rhythm showed on the screen. I checked for a pulse. "I have a pulse!"

"I hope it will stay this time," said John. The patient was still not breathing on his own. John bagged him, while I hooked the oxygen to the bag mask. I looked back at the monitor and saw the heart rate was forty bpm. Sixty bpm is the slowest speed that was safe. If it went any lower, not enough oxygenated blood would reach the brain.

"I'll get the atropine," I said, reaching into the drug box. I grabbed an amp and pushed the dose into the IV. "Atropine on board." I felt the pulse. It was slow and weak, but it was there. The heart rate started to pick up some speed.

"Rate is at fifty," I told John. Then shortly after, "Rate is at sixty." I checked his blood pressure and it was 100/60 which was very good for this patient.

By the time I was done taking the blood pressure, we were at the hospital. While enroute I had been writing down all the drugs and times given on the incident report. I also noted all the defib's and times administered. All the ECG's were stored on the LIFEPAK computer for me to print when needed.

We pulled the patient out of the Rescue and into the ER while John was still bagging him. We were met by a nurse who ushered us into a cardiac care room. The doctor and nurses cleaned him up and put in a subclavian line. The doctor turned to us and said, "You guys did a great job."

"Thank you, doc," we replied. It was nice getting a compliment once and a while. As we left, I said to John, "It was a good save, but I don't think he will walk out of here."

"Yeah, you're probably right," John replied.

The reason I remembered this run was because it was so unusual. First: the patient kept trying to get up. People in cardiac arrest just don't do that, but he did. That's what confused us at the scene and made us initially not believe that he was really in cardiac arrest. We were able to reach the patient only a minute or two after he arrested.

Second: It almost never happens that a person in systole can ever come back. But he did. One theory is he may have been in very fine fib, which could explain it. Anyway, I had never seen those things before or since. And to make it even more amazing, the patient walked out of the hospital a week or two later.

When John and I finished the reports, we picked up the replacement drugs from the hospital pharmacy and went back to Station Four just in time for dinner. We were having donkey dicks, salad and smashed taters for dinner. Everyone at the department affectionately called Polish sausage 'donkey dicks.' We had crazy nicknames for a lot of things.

At the dinner table we talked about the cardiac arrest case and the crazy things that had happened. Everyone shared their theories about why it had happened the way it did. Somehow the conversation switched to chronic callers. Some were lonely housewives. Some were old men or women that craved attention.

Then there was Mr. Hodges, a man of about eighty years old. We went to his house almost every day, because he was worried about his blood pressure way too much. We would go over and he would be worried that his blood pressure was too low or too high. Everyone knew where he lived without looking the address up.

One day we went there, and Mr. Hodges was sitting in his recliner like he always was. His son was there to bring him a new blood pressure cuff because he wore the last one out. The son noticed that we knew his dad by name.

"You've been here before," he commented.

"Yes, sir, we have checked in on him many times."

"He takes his blood pressure so many times a day, I can't keep track," the son said.

I said to him and his father, "You know, it doesn't help to take your blood pressure so many times. In fact, it makes you worry. When you worry, your blood pressure goes up and you worry more. It's a vicious cycle."

"Yes," Mr. Hodges responded, "I know. I will try to take my blood pressure less and worry less, I promise."

We were back there later that same evening. We couldn't not go, because that would be the time that he was really in trouble.

John looked across the table and asked me, "Do you remember Mrs. Mink?"

"Oh yes, Mrs. Mink," I answered. "I haven't run on her for a long time."

Now, John was a great story teller. Even though sometimes it took him forever to get to the point, everyone was captivated along the way. "Mrs.

Mink," John mused. "We used to go to her house most every day once we had our first run there."

"One afternoon," John started, "we were dispatched to do a welfare check at her house on Sunset Avenue. Mrs. Mink's son had not heard from her yet that day and she always called him.

It was just Greg and me on this run. We parked the squad in her driveway and knocked on the door. No one answered. If she had, that would be the end of the story. But she didn't.

Two large white poodles glared at us through the glass door, showing their teeth. We waited for a bit, and then tried the door. It was locked. We walked around the house, trying the other doors, but they were all locked tight. We found an open window leading to the kitchen, above the sink. G.J. climbed in and onto the sink counter. The dogs were barking and snarling below."

I took over the story at that point. "I climbed down off the sink and the two tough watch dogs whined, ran away and hid. Meanwhile, I realized that I had landed in a pile of dog poop." That got a laugh from the guys.

"I went to the front door and let John in. There was dog poop everywhere. We had to maneuver around the piles like a mine field."

John jumped in. "We heard a muffled sound coming from up the stairs. We went up and the sound became louder, but it was still muted, like the speaker's head was covered. However, it was clear that someone was calling for help from the bedroom. When we walked in, she was nowhere to be seen.

"I yelled, 'Is anyone here?' A voice from somewhere near the bed said, 'I am beside the bed and I'm stuck!' The bed was against the wall. We went to the end of it, and there she was, a sixty year-old woman wedged between the wall and the bed. She was a heavy-set woman with humungous breasts. She said these words that I will never forget. 'Get this off my face!'

I took over the story telling again. "John said, 'get what off your face?' 'I can't breathe! My breast is on my face and I can't move!' Apparently, she had slipped off the bed and became stuck against the wall. While she was struggling, she somehow got her very large breast draped over her face. So she was stuck like that until we found her. 'Please get this off my face. I can't breathe.'"

"Lucky for me, John hadn't been promoted yet and I had more seniority," I commented.

John spoke up. "It took both hands to lift the giant breast off her face, and it went 'slap!' when it landed on the floor. We got her out by moving the bed and helped her back onto it. After that we were there every day for a long time."

"She had a crush on you, John," I teased as the story ended. No sooner had we finished telling the story than we got a run.

"Station Three and Rescue Four, you have a lady lying on the floor of her house with severe abdominal pain at 4444 Fallow. Time out, 1922."

"Fallow is off Green Lake Road," Lt. Bigger told us. "Rescue Four responding," someone called in.

"Engine Three responding." The lieutenant decided to stay back this time. Marty rode shot gun instead.

"Responding received, Engine Three and Rescue Four."

Fallow was on the other side of Station Three, which meant we had to drive past their station to reach the address. "Engine Three on scene," they called in.

"On scene received, Engine Three."

With our lights and siren blaring, we were able to shoot through traffic easily. There were no medics at Station Three that day, so we needed to get there as soon as possible. We arrived a few minutes after Engine Three. I pulled up behind their vehicle while Marty called, "Rescue Four on scene."

I was concerned because I had dealt with a patient with a dissecting descending aortic aneurysm not very long ago that acted much like the run we were heading to. It ruptured before we could get there, and the patient died right in front of us. There was absolutely nothing we could do.

A descending aortic artery is the largest artery in your body, descending from your heart down to your legs. An aneurysm is like a bike tire bulging out of the rim. It makes a bubble that, if not operated on in time, will burst open and almost instantly kill a person by causing them to bleed to death internally. So I was in a hurry. I don't ever want to see that again.

We hurried with the equipment to the front door. Bob opened it for us. As I entered the house, I could smell the unpleasant fragrance of vomit in the air. There, in front of us, was a young lady in her early twenties. She was curled up on the floor in a fetal position and was crying in pain. Marty asked her mother what had happened as we knelt down beside the patient.

"Did you see her fall?" Marty asked.

The mom answered in a shaky voice, "She was getting ready to go to night school. She screamed and I saw her fall and curl up into a ball. Then she vomited."

To make it even worse for the young lady, she was lying in the vomit and had it caked in her beautiful blond hair. I asked the girl, "Where is your pain?"

"It's everywhere!" She screamed, clearly in agony. "On a scale of one to ten for the pain, what...?"

She cut me off, yelling, "Ten! Ten! Tennnn!" She was distressed and cried out, "I'm dying! I'm dying!"

We all knew what she had just by looking at her. I said, "You are not dying. I have some good news and some bad news. The good news is you have kidney stones. The bad news is you will be in pain until the stone passes."

I have seen kidney stones many times. Most people say it is the most painful thing they have ever experienced. We often find kidney stone patients rolled up in a ball on the floor. It strikes suddenly.

We cleaned the patient up, and when the ambulance arrived, we handed her over to the advanced crew. There wasn't anything more we could do for her. Marty called it in to the hospital, and they would not allow her to have anything for pain. She just needed transportation to the hospital. We assured her and her mother that she was going to be just fine.

The ambulance left with the mother following behind in her car. We always warned the families of a patient that follow behind the ambulance not to drive too closely, and not to go through a red light just because the ambulance does.

"Engine Three and Rescue Four in service, returning to quarters," Bob called from Engine Three.

"In service, returning received, Engine Three and Rescue Four."

We got about a mile away when the tones went off. "Station Four, a possible PIA at the intersection of Commerce Road and Hiller. Time out, 2022."

"Engine Three, Rescue Four responding."

"Responding received." It only took about two minutes to get to the intersection.

"Engine Three and Rescue Four on scene." I pulled Rescue Four right behind a lone car in the middle of the intersection, stopped directly beneath the traffic light. Engine Three had blocked the intersection so no vehicles could interfere with us at the scene. In the car we found a woman slumped behind the steering wheel.

The first thing I noticed was that there was no damage to the car and it was still in drive. I put the car in park and turned off the engine. Then I felt for a pulse.

"I have a pulse and she's breathing." As we were assessing the patient, the police arrived and directed traffic.

"It looks like low blood sugar," Marty announced.

"I think you're right," I said in agreement. Marty had the clipboard, so I got out the blood test strips and lance. I quickly poked her finger and touched the blood to the test strip.

"Her blood glucose is twenty," I said. Twenty is very low. Usually when the blood glucose level, is that low it is because the patient took insulin and did not eat enough. Although, in the case of brittle diabetics, they often have trouble keeping their blood sugar stable at any time.

"I'm going to start an IV and give a vial of glucose." I started the IV and pushed the amp of glucose into the tube. It takes a minute or two to administer because the amp is so large, about an inch and a half in diameter. That's a lot to get through the IV tube. But once the amp is on board, it is like magic.

Almost immediately after giving the glucose, the patient woke up. She was confused for a short time, but then she asked, "What happened?"

"You had low blood sugar," I answered. "You passed out in the middle of the intersection."

"I did?" she asked. "Oh now I remember. I felt weak and I called my husband. Then things went dark. I think he is on his way."

"As we speak, here he is," I told her, noticing a worried looking man approaching the car. By that time, she was alert and wanted to get up. Her husband wanted to take her home.

"She is fine and I want her home."

"Ok," I said. "Let us get her vitals and call the hospital first."

Her blood pressure was good. She was alert and she wanted to go home. Marty called the hospital and they advised for her husband to drive her home.

"Ok," Marty said. "The doctor said you can take her home, but you have to drive."

"Park the car in the gas station parking lot while I take out the IV," I suggested.

I took out the IV and they went home. With diabetics, they usually know what's happening because they've been through it before, and when they are given dextrose and wake up, they don't want any more help. They also know that we can't force them to go to the ER.

"Rescue Four at quarters, finally," Marty called as the apparatus room doors closed.

"Rescue Four at quarters, finally," repeated Dispatch.

I turned off the truck and went into the living room, sat on the recliner and watched some mind-numbing TV. After a while, I hit the sack, knowing I needed to rest when I could, because you never knew what was coming next.

# Chapter 26 - On the Run

Getting a run while you're sound asleep could be unsettling. That night, I was jolted out of sleep by the thunder of the tones and the crash of the bright bunk room lights. I worked at so many different stations, that it always took me a few seconds to remember where I was when awoken like that.

"Station Four, Station Three, you have a structure fire at 9765 Greer, next door to the German park. Flames visible."

It seemed so painful to me to be startled awake like that. From zero to one hundred in an instant. We all popped out of our bunks and hopped into our bunker pants. We met at the watch desk, got the assignment, then went out the door to our vehicles.

"Engine Four, Rescue Four responding," Lieutenant called from the Engine passenger seat.

"Engine Three and Tanker Three responding," Bob called from Engine Three.

"Responding received, Engine Three, Tanker Three, Engine Four, Rescue Four."

"Engine One, Ladder One, Captain's car responding," we heard from Station One across the township.

"Responding received, Engine One, Ladder One, Captain's car."

During all that radio chatter, I noticed the brightly lit sky. We were still a mile away, but we could see the flames from there. I don't remember if there were any hydrants, but even if there were, they'd be unreliable at best. I did not get the chance to find out.

As we pulled up, I saw an attached garage with flames raging out of the roof into the night sky. Sparks streaked up along with black smoke, bellowing skyward. Marty was in the back, putting on his air pack. I took my air pack out of the side compartment and put it on. I was getting ready to pull hose off the Engine, when I saw someone lying in the snow in front of the garage.

Marty and I got closer and saw an unconscious man lying face down in the snow. The lieutenant was calling us to pull the hose out. I picked up my hand radio and spoke to him. "Lieutenant, we have a man down in the snow in front of the garage."

"Ok, Rescue Four, I will get someone else. Take care of him." Marty reached the patient first and turned him over. I knelt down beside him. I could see by the color of his face that he was not breathing. He had a garden hose in his hand, the water still running out of it.

"He's in cardiac arrest," Marty said. A working fire with a cardiac arrest out in front. If that doesn't get your heart rate up, I don't know what will.

While kneeling there, glowing embers started dropping around us. It was very hot and getting hotter. The tree that we were under was catching on fire too. "We'd better move him!" I yelled to Marty. "Let's take him to the Rescue."

Engine Three had just arrived. They helped us pick the old man up out of the snow and carry him to the Rescue. It was a mess in the back, where we had prepped to help with the fire. I hopped into the back and cleared the stretcher of all of the stray equipment. Then we placed the patient onto the stretcher.

I opened his airway and confirmed that he wasn't breathing. I checked for a pulse and found none. "He's cold to the touch," I told the others. I opened his coat and ripped open his shirt.

Over the radio, I heard, "Engine One, Captain one on scene."

Bob opened the back and asked, "Do you want me to drive?"

"Yes, that would be great!" Marty answered. Bob got in front and we took off. We bounced around in back while Bob maneuvered the Rescue out. Marty grabbed the quick-look paddles. The monitor showed a-systole. Straight line.

The man was ninety, and we knew he had no chance, but we had to try. Marty pulled his own coat off while I got out the bag mask and started ventilating the patient. Marty started an IV, but it took a few tries because the patient's skin was cold from being outside.

When he got the IV in I told him, "Good job! That was a hard one." Marty set up the ECG while I intubated the patient. He was still in a-systole and remained flat line until we got to the hospital.

They pronounced him dead not too long after we arrived. We used the whole drug box treating him on the way in, but he was DRT (dead right there) at the scene. He never had a chance.

We surmised that he had been working in his garage and somehow started the fire. He must have gotten excited and ran around to get the garden hose to put out the flames, but had a heart attack and was DRT. We ran the code on him anyway, but we knew he wouldn't make it. I supposed it was always possible, but I had never seen anyone that was in a-systole when we arrived survive.

We did the report and picked up the replacement drugs. By the time we left the hospital, it was after shift change. It was 0830 when we entered the township.

Marty called, "Rescue Four in service in the township and heading back to the fire."

"Engine Four to Rescue Four, return to quarters. We have it wrapped up here."

"Ok, returning to Station Four."

"Returning to quarters, received, Rescue Four."

Marty complained all the way back to the station that we missed a good hot working garage and house fire.

Time passed quickly, overall. I enjoyed my time off with my family; I stayed busy and tried to keep fit. Although I had the most seniority in the department of any non-officer, I was still shuffled from one station to another if there wasn't an officer on duty that day. Yes, I got a little extra "in-charge" pay, but I would have rather been able to stay at my own station. Station Four was one I was assigned to for quite a while.

"Station Four, a snowmobile accident at 1896 Horas. Time out, 2130. Be advised that the snowmobile accident is behind the residence on the lake and someone may be trapped in the water."

It just so happened that we had been drilling on cold water rescue, so we were ready. I was driving the Engine that day. Meanwhile, in the back of the Rescue, the boys were prepping the ice water rescue gear. The apparatus room doors opened and off we went into the night.

I thought it looked oddly pretty, with the red lights reflecting off the snow as we raced to a possible injury or drowning on a lake. We knew that the address was near the Chief's house. Sure enough, the Chief was outside when we arrived.

"Engine Four, Rescue on scene," we called in. The Chief met us as we got out of our trucks. He pointed
out to the open darkness of the lake where the snowmobile crash had occurred.

The lieutenant asked the Chief, "Is the ice safe to walk on?"

"Yes," he said, "It's plenty thick near shore. It's just that there is a spring out there and the ice didn't freeze this winter."

The boys from the Rescue came over with their orange ice rescue suits. I got mine out of the side compartment, and the lieutenant put an orange life vest on. We got out the Stokes stretcher, some rope, flashlights and other equipment and headed toward the lake, pulling the gear in the basket behind us.

The Chief said, "It's about one hundred yards over there, at the tree line. There is a point of land jutting out into the water." He gestured out towards the lake.

We dragged the equipment out to the area where the chief had indicated. The lieutenant shined the light out over the general area. There was a figure moving across the dark snow. He was yelling, but we couldn't hear what he was trying to say. As the man reached us, he stopped, panting and out of breath.

He told us, "Our snowmobile fell through the ice and is sinking. Please save our snowmobile."

Lieutenant asked, "Is anyone hurt?"

"No," the guy replied, "but my snowmobile is sinking!"

We followed him to a big hole in the ice, about fifty feet across. A snowmobile was floating in the water. "What happened?" I asked.

"We were riding, having a good time, when all of the sudden, the two of us flew over the snowmobile as it hit the water. We landed on the other side of the ice hole."

"You flew all that way and no one is hurt?"

"Yeah, we landed in the soft snow." He put his arm around the lady he was with. We got the rope out and were going to attach it to the machine, when lights appeared in the distance, rapidly approaching. I could hear the unmistakable sound of a snowmobile engine.

We all watched in shock as two snowmobiles came barreling in our direction. We shined our flash lights at them, trying to signal, but it didn't work. They flew past us, a plume of snow streaking out behind them. Both snowmobiles splashed into the water, and came to a sudden stop as they hit the side of the ice.

The two people on each vehicle flew over the top of the snow- mobiles and landed on the other side in a poof of soft snow, then slid about ten feet further and came to a stop. It was just like what the first guy had described. We ran toward the riders, reaching them just as they were getting themselves up.

"Is everyone all right?" Lieutenant asked.

They brushed the snow off for a second and nodded their heads. "Ok, I guess."

We all walked back to the hole in the ice.

"We were just going for a ride. All of a sudden we were flying through the air," one man said.

They were all talking at once and that assured us they were all right. Lieutenant asked if anyone needed to be looked at, but they all refused treatment. No one even had a scratch. Now there were three snowmobiles in the hole in the ice. "Please help me get my snowmobile out of the water!" the first man begged, but it was too late. It had already sunk.

"Rescue Four, you can return to quarters while we put markers out," said Lieutenant. We put emergency tape out around the hole, but it didn't matter. Two more snowmobiles fell through the ice that night. They just couldn't see well enough until it was too late.

We all arrived back at the station at about midnight. I left the lieutenant to finish his reports and went to bed. We were all able to sleep the rest of the night.

The next day I was working at Station Three, and I was in charge. In fact I had just received my promotion to Sergeant. I was in charge of one guy, Mike. It had been raining all morning, and the temperature was dropping rapidly. The roads were going be a mess. The tones went off.

"Station Three and Rescue Four, respond to a possible suicide at 3576 Bennett. No other information available. Time out, 0922."

We went to the watch desk, looked up the address and headed out the door to our truck. Mike was driving, and I was in the passenger seat. We drove out the apparatus door and turned right.

"Engine Three responding," I called into the mic. "Take this fork in the road to the left, It's the third house on the right," I directed Mike. We stopped in front of a small two-story house.

"Engine Three on scene." We took the first aid kit from the side compartment and hurried up to the front door.

"Engine Three from dispatch, be advised that the call came from a concerned family member not at this residence. She said that she got a call from her ex and that he said he was going to kill himself."

"Message received," I confirmed.

We were at the front door. Mike said, "I'll kick open the door."

I put my hand on the door knob, twisted it and the door opened. Always check for an unlocked door before knocking it down was the lesson for Mike to learn here. As we entered, I saw a stairway right in front of us.

"Let's go up first," I suggested. Mike was already running up the stairs. When he reached top he said.

"He's here! Up here!" When I got to the room, Mike was trying to lift a man that had a rope around his neck. The rope stretched up to a beam in the ceiling. I hurried to help Mike take the man's weight off the rope. I got out my knife and cut it. We slowly eased him down to the floor. He was lifeless and stiff.

The man was about forty years old. There was dried drool extending from his mouth and down his chin. The man's face was a dark gray color. "He's been here for a while," I said to Mike as Officer Miller entered the house.

"Where are you?" Miller called.

"Upstairs," I shouted back. Officer Miller and another officer ran to the top of the stairs and looked for a moment.

The other officer said, "Why did you cut him down?"

"We had to!" Mike snapped defensively. "We didn't know if he was alive or not."

"You disturbed a possible crime scene," complained the officer.

"We did what we had to do!" Mike yelled back. Mike liked confrontation and was eager to argue with the officer. I have to admit I enjoyed watching Mike in combat.

Rescue Four arrived and that ended the argument for a while. We met the crew of the Rescue at the top of the stairs. "He's been here for a long time," Joe from Rescue Four said.

"He is also cold to the touch," I said. "He's been hanging here for twelve hours or less."

The man had rigor mortis, which meant he was stiff. The muscles and joints get inflexible not too long after a person dies. After about twelve hours the body starts to relax again. So, if the body is not stiff anymore, you know the person has been dead for longer than twelve hours.

The other officer was still copping an attitude with us, but Joe told him, "We have to call it in to the hospital and get a TOD (time of death). And we have to send an ECG strip to the hospital to confirm."

To Mike and I, Joe said, "We have this. Engine Three can head back." Mike always had to have the last word. As we walked away, he told the officer, "Make yourself useful and call the ME."

"Engine Three in service," I called to Dispatch as I grabbed Mike by the shirt and led him down the stairs.

We were barely back in the vehicle when we got our next call. "Engine Three, Rescue One, respond to a child having trouble breathing at 3496 Hiller Wood."

We rushed to the Engine knowing that Rescue would not be able to respond until the hanging case was complete. Rescue One would have to respond instead. The address was behind Station Three, so we headed in that direction.

"Engine Three responding," I called into the mic as I flipped on the emergency lights. I looked up the address on the map. We got there in less than two minutes. As we arrived I told Mike, "As soon as we stop, I will run in. You bring the equipment."

I called, "Engine Three on scene," as I ran to the door of a large house. The door flew open and I rushed in.

A woman yelled, "My baby can't breathe! He's with my husband in the bathroom."

I heard some coughing, which sounded like seal barks. I knew what that sound meant. She led me to the bathroom and opened the door. A cloud of steam rolled out. I entered the warm room, and through the thick steam I saw a man holding a two year old boy.

I said, "I'm from the Fire Department. It sounds like your son has croup."

Then he said to me, "He has been coughing like this all day. It has been getting a lot worse. I have had him in this steam for about fifteen minutes, and he hasn't gotten any better."

Usually, croup is not too dangerous. But sometimes it can become life-threatening if not taken care of. You can identify croup because the cough sounds like a seal barking. To new parents, it can be terrifying. He cried, "This is not working! I am doing what the book says to do!"

"Let me try something," I suggested. I held my arms out and he handed the baby to me. The baby was coughing almost constantly. I took him out of the steamy bathroom, the new father following close behind me.

I talked as I walked, "If steam doesn't work, try something else. We need a new setting." I opened the front door and took the baby outside into the cold. "If warm steam doesn't work, try the opposite. Dry cold."

Within a minute, the baby stopped coughing. I gave him back to his father as Rescue One arrived. The boy was already asleep. I gave the low down to the Rescue One crew for their paperwork. The parents declined transport to the hospital.

"Engine Three can go back to quarters." That statement was always music to my ears. At Station Three, I had to finish the paperwork for the runs before I went to bed. I got the coffee ready and on the timer for morning before I turned in. We slept well for a while, until about 0730.

# Chapter 27 - Endings and Beginnings

"Engine Three and Rescue Two, respond to a PIA at Pontiac Trail and Haggerty Road. A reported head-on collision. Time out, 0734. Be advised the roads are very slippery."

The dorm lights burned my eyes as I struggled to shake off sleep. Brushing that feeling aside, I went to the watch room where Mike was already waiting. We ran to the trucks in our gear, pushed the door opener and climbed into Engine Three. It just so happened that Tim, from the other unit, came in early.

"Tim," I called, "you can take the pickup." We pulled out of the apparatus room doors with Utility Three following some ways behind. "Take it slow with the ice on the road," I cautioned.
We turned out onto Green Lake Road and I called to Dispatch, "Engine Three and Utility Three responding."

"Responding received, all units." The light was just beginning to brighten the morning. The head lights and red overhead lights reflected off the ice on the road. I felt the tires slip a little.

"Careful," I cautioned. "Better to get there late than not at all." Tim must have seen us slide a little because he called us.

"Engine Three, be careful up there. You fish-tailed a little."

Even though we had slowed some, it still was a white-knuckle trip. We took Green Lake to Pontiac Trail and turned right. It was a clear shot from there to the intersection of Pontiac Trail and Haggerty. Pontiac Trail was a narrow two-lane road with ditches on either side. Scattered houses lined the road.

About a mile down, we fish-tailed again before straightening out. Then, the rear of our Engine started sliding. Suddenly there was no control. I felt the ten-ton Engine skid.

I knew this would be bad, so I pushed back in my seat, bracing for impact. The rear of the Engine passed the front and we started to spin. I could see field, then the road, then the field again as we made a 360.

We slid most the way around and were now facing back the way we had come, but the Engine was still sliding. We followed the contour of the sloping road toward the ditch. I knew if we struck the ditch, we would flip.

We hit the shoulder sideways, snow and mud blowing into the air. We bounced off the shoulder and slid past the ditch into a field, still facing the way we had been headed. Then we came to a dead stop. We didn't flip.

Nothing was said for a long moment. Utility Three broke the silence. "Are you guys ok in there?" That was Tim, who had watched the whole thing.

"We're fine, Tim," I answered. "Continue on to the PIA. We will be there as soon as we can." I looked out the window and saw the reason we didn't flip. Our tires had found an old abandoned driveway and slid right over the ditch.

There were two fifteen-foot long sideways slide divots from the road to the shoulder to where we were now resting in a field. I don't know how we found the driveway, but we did. I can only say that God was looking out for us. If we would have tipped over, we could have been crushed. The cab does not provide much protection for that kind of weight.

After a moment, I calmly said to Mike, "We still have a PIA to go to."

Mike's hands were shaking and so were mine. I didn't realize how close we came to tipping over until I went to the slide site the next day. Mike maneuvered the truck back over the old driveway and onto the road. I didn't have to tell my driver this time to go slower. Engine Three was the last one to get to the PIA, but at least we got there safely.

There was construction along Haggerty. They were black topping the two lane road, and it still needed another coat. There were manholes sticking out of the road about eight inches high. With the next coat of asphalt, they would be flush.

We saw two destroyed cars, about ten feet apart, in the intersection. Police had blocked traffic. Rescue Two was already treating the possible injuries. "Engine Three on scene," I said as we stopped.

The cars were a mess, and they both had their air bags deployed. There was no one in the cars. I had Mike pull out the rolled one-inch hose to the front of the accident. There probably wasn't going to be a fire, but I couldn't take the chance. I walked over to the Rescue Two crew to see where the patients were.

"Over by the police car," I was told. There were two men talking to the police. It turned out that one of the drivers hit the manhole in the road and lost control of his car. He crossed over the center line and crashed head-on into the second car. The only injuries were mild face burns caused by the airbags deploying. The airbags saved both their lives without a doubt.

We reeled up the hose and headed back to Station Three, but we didn't make it. Along the way, we got another call. "Engine Three, welfare check at 4445 Crescent Road. A man called and said his daughter won't answer her phone. He says he calls her every morning. Time out, 0755."

"Engine Three responding."

"Responding received. Be advised the lady is a diabetic." The house was a small old box house with no garage. A car was parked in the driveway.

"Engine Three on scene," I called in. We walked up to the front door and found it unlocked. I knocked, but no one answered. I opened the door and called out, "Fire Department!" Still no answer.

I saw an open door in front of us. As I entered, I noticed another door leading to a bedroom. We walked in and found a slim lady of about thirty lying on the bed with the covers over her legs, wearing a tiny nighty. She looked as if she was asleep.

"Ma'am! Ma'am!" I called, but she didn't move. I went over to her to wake her, placing my hand on her shoulder. Her skin was ice cold. I then lifted up her hand and her whole arm came up. She was as stiff as a board. I picked the hand radio mic from my lapel and called, "Engine Three to Dispatch. We will need Rescue Two and a patrol car here. We have a DOS (dead on scene)."

Then the phone rang. I picked up the phone, knowing it was going to be her father. "Hello, this is Sergeant Johnson with the West Bloomfield Fire Department."

"Ah, this is John Hill. Is my daughter alright?"

"Mr. Hill, I'm sorry to have to tell you that she expired during the night," I sadly told him. He told me that she was a divorced, thirty year-old lady that lived alone. She was a brittle diabetic. He had been worried about this happening, and that's why he called her every morning. It was a sad day for her family, no doubt.

The police arrived, followed a short time later by Rescue Two. There was nothing more we could do, so we headed back to the station to go home.

The years flew by. The kids grew up, and I was getting older. I thought after twenty years of being a paramedic that it was time to let the youngsters take over the medicals. As a result, I decided to give up my medical license.

You might think that would be the end of medical runs for me, but it made no difference. I just didn't have to start IV's or suction vomit.

Shortly after I gave up my license, I had the most important medical run of my career. I was again stationed at Station Three. John was with me that day. The morning had hardly begun when the tones went off.

"Station Three and Rescue Four, respond to a child with something caught in his throat at 5998 Knight Bridge Lane. The father says he is not breathing. He is being instructed in CPR. Time out, 0922. Be advised I have a patrol car dispatched."

Having children myself, I could not imagine the terror that those parents were now going through. John and I hurried to the Engine. We shot out from the apparatus room door, with lights and sirens blaring. We headed south on Green Lake Road. I was driving this time, and I didn't have to say anything about the urgency. We had a four-to-six minute window before brain injury would occur.

As we barreled down the two-lane street, all the cars in either direction pulled off to the shoulder and got out of the way. I realized that Rescue Four was going to have to pass by Station Three to get to the scene. That meant they would be at least two minutes behind us, so it was up to John and me.

The thought came to mind that I had been lucky not to have any serous medicals on children since having my own children. I knew it would be devastating for me to lose one now.

It seemed to take forever to get to the scene. Just before we got there, John said to me, "When we get there, you go on in and I will get the equipment."

I nodded my head and calmly said, "Ok, John." I had to keep myself composed because I would have to be able to think quickly and clearly.

But on the other hand, like so many choking runs before, maybe by the time we got to the scene the object in his throat would already be dislodged.

"Engine Three on scene," I stopped the rig in front of the house, put it in park and quickly pulled on the air brake. I opened the door and ran to the front of the house. I yanked the door open and yelled, "Fire Department!"

"In here!" was the reply. "We're in here!" A quivering woman's voice screamed. I ran into the living room and found a woman carrying a limp toddler in her arms. "He swallowed a grape!" She hysterically screamed. "He has a grape stuck in his throat!" She handed me the unconscious four year old.

I took the lifeless, tiny body in my arms. His legs draped over my forearms. His small face was blue in color, and he was not breathing.

"He has a grape stuck in his throat!" the mother cried again. I took the boy and draped him face down over my arm and sharply patted his back to dislodge the grape. Four blows on his back.

I turned him over to check the airway. The little blue face was still not breathing. I turned him back over and delivered four more blows to his back with no effect. By this time, John had entered the house with the equipment. The gear he had was going to do me no good unless we could clear the airway.

I sharply patted the young boy's back four more times. I turned him up again, but he still had whatever it was stuck in his throat. I had a very low sinking feeling in my stomach as I peered into his dull eyes. I paused for a moment, realizing that the training I took for this crisis was not going to work. This young boy's life was passing away while he was in my arms, because I couldn't get the grape out.

By then, the Rescue Four crew had come in with all their equipment. I set the small body down on the floor to try something else. I was trained not to put my finger in a victim's throat as a method to try to dislodge a foreign object, because you can push it in further.

Well, this boy was going to die, if he wasn't already dead, if I didn't get the object out now! I stuck my finger as deep into his throat as I could reach, knowing that this would most likely not work either. I felt something on the tip of my finger. I managed to reach a little deeper and put my finger around something. I pulled my finger out and a grape popped out as well, falling onto the floor.

"I got it out!" I said in disbelief. "Is he breathing?" John asked.

"No," I answered as I checked his mouth. I opened his airway and did mouth to mouth. I covered his mouth and nose with my mouth and puffed air into his lungs. At the same time I felt for a pulse. The Rescue crew was setting up the LIFEPAK and IV as I checked for a pulse. I felt a wave of relief as I found one.

"He has a pulse!" I said excitedly. I looked down at the small face and noticed he had blood coming out of his mouth. I didn't worry about the blood just then, and I gave him some more mouth to mouth breaths.

Officer Cooper had arrived by then. I don't know when he got there, but suddenly he was offering to help. I asked him, "Can you do mouth to mouth?"

"I think so, but I've only practiced on adult manikins." "Ok, I will help you," I assured him.

"He has blood coming out of his mouth," Officer Cooper pointed out, seemingly reluctant.

"Don't worry about that now, he's a child," I told him firmly.

Officer Cooper put his mouth over the child's mouth.

"Not too much air," I instructed him. "About half of what you would give to an adult."

He gave ventilations as I checked the pulse again. "The pulse is stronger!" I said. The child's color was a lot better, so I told the officer to stop mouth to mouth for a ten count.

"He is breathing!" I said excitedly. The breathing was weak but it was there. The Rescue crew was ready to take over now, so I handed him over to Bob.

"We've got this now," he said. "We will start the IV in the Rescue." He rushed out the door with the baby. The other two from the Rescue followed, carrying equipment.

John and I helped carry out the rest of the gear to the Rescue so they could leave right away. I placed the last of the items in the back of the truck and closed the door.

I watched as Rescue Four, with lights flashing, disappeared around the corner. Even though the Rescue was out of sight, I still heard the sound of the siren in the distance. And then they were gone.

I turned back to the house and passed John carrying our own equipment back to Engine Three. "I have to talk to the parents," I said to John.

Officer Cooper was walking toward me. I asked him, "Can you ask the dispatcher for me how long it took
for us to get here and what time Rescue Four left? That should tell me how long he went without air."
"Sure," he replied, "I can do that." He reached for his lapel mic.

"Thanks," I said, walking back into the house. I hadn't noticed that the father had gone in the Rescue with the child. When I entered the house, the mother was sitting on a stool in the kitchen, crying.

I tried to reassure her, saying, "I got the grape out and he was breathing when he left."

"But Joey was not breathing for such a long, long time!" she cried. The officer came in and waved me over.

"About seven minutes we figure he was down," Officer Cooper reported to me.

"Thanks," I responded, "I will tell her." I went back into the kitchen and told her, "Joey is very young and he was without air for about seven minutes. Young children can handle seven minutes without oxygen where adults can't. Of course, I can't promise anything, but I think he will be alright."

I patted her on the back. Then she put her arms around me to hug me and started crying. I put my arms around her and stood there until she was ready to leave for the hospital.

She said, "Thank you," then let me go, picked up her things and went to her car. Now everyone was gone but us. John locked the front door and said, "Engine Three is in service."

It was over now, and I should have felt good, but I didn't. I told John on the way back, "I don't know if we did the family or Joey any good. He probably will have some brain damage if he even lives." I added, "And I don't know. Maybe I gave the mother false hope."

"Engine Three at quarters," John called.

"Engine Three at quarters, received." As I got out of the Engine, the phone rang. John picked up the receiver, shook his head, then handed it to me.

"Hello?" I said into the phone.

"I heard you had a good save of a four year old." It was the officer in charge of emergency medical services for the Department.

"Well," I said, "he was alive at the time he left the house."

"He is at the hospital now and is breathing on his own, so good save," he said to me.

"I only hope we didn't burden the family more by keeping him alive with brain damage," I said. "We figure he was without oxygen for at least seven minutes."

"Nothing you can do about what happens before and after you were there," he told me. "The only thing you have to think about is that you did a good job on the save."

He added, "It's funny that you had one of the most important medicals of your career when you were no longer a medic."

"Yeah, it is kind of ironic," I agreed.

"Any way, I heard that you may have gotten some blood in your mouth on the medical."

"Yes," I admitted. "He was bleeding from his mouth, probably from when I pulled the grape out. Officer Cooper did mouth to mouth as well."

"Why didn't you use a bag mask?" he asked me.

I replied, "because he is just a baby and I needed to ventilate him quickly and efficiently. The bag mask would have taken too long."

"Well," he said, "it turned out well, except," he paused for a moment, "you will have to go to the hospital right away and get a blood test because of the exposure. So hop in the pickup and drive yourself to the hospital right away. Fill out a blood exposure report when you get back."

"Ok," I said.

"Good job," he told me as he hung up the phone.

"Well, John, I have to go to the hospital and get a blood test," I said. "I'm sure Joey's blood is clean, but the rules are you get a blood test with an exposure."

I remember when I first started in my career. We didn't even know about blood-borne pathogens. We started IV's with no gloves on. On traumas we got covered in blood and thought nothing of it. That is until AIDS came along. Then we became aware of hepatitis as well. After that, we wore gloves for everything.

I hopped in the pickup and headed to the hospital. It was a long wait in the emergency room for me. About four hours later, after getting my blood tested, I was about to leave the ER when I spotted Joey and his mother behind a curtain, still in a room.

Joey was unconscious, lying on the gurney, his eyes taped shut. His mother was holding his hand, looking at him with sad eyes. That sight hit me like a ton of bricks. I felt pain like I had never felt before. I walked a little past the curtain so she couldn't see me. I stood there for a few minutes, trying to decide if I should talk to her
or not. A doctor was about to enter the room. I stopped him before he went in.

"How is he?" I asked.

"Who wants to know?" he challenged.

"I was on the run with him," I responded. "I did mouth to mouth on him."

The doctor nodded and said, "he is very young. He should be alright in a few days."

"He was without oxygen for seven or so minutes," I protested.

"He could have brain damage, but young brains are resilient," the doctor reassured me. "He will probably be ok, but mentally he may be knocked down a few pegs." He then turned to walk into the room. I had started feeling better about myself after the call from the medical director.

After seeing Joey and his mom, then talking to the doctor, I felt terrible. I later found out that Joey's blood was clean, but I would still have to get a series of blood tests anyway. What a pain. I knew it was for my own safety, but it was still a pain.

When I got back to the station, I didn't feel like doing much. That run affected me like no other. I don't remember what happened the rest of the shift or even the rest of the week.

The next week I had to report to Station One for the paperwork and then take it to the hospital for another blood test. It was morning when I arrived at Station One.

One of the men had just been out getting bagels. The Captain offered me one while I was waiting for the paper work. I was still feeling very low and I guess it showed. Normally, the others would joke with me, but now everyone left me alone.

I picked up a bagel and proceeded to cut it in half with a serrated knife. As I was sawing the bagel, the blade cut deep into my finger. I had never done that before. I guess I just wasn't thinking clearly.

The guys got me bandages to clean up my wound. It was cut clear to the bone, and I was going to need some stitches. There was blood on the table and the floor.

The men helped me clean up the mess and didn't say a word about my debacle. It was hard enough with the way I was feeling. I didn't need to be teased by the guys now, and they, sensing this, didn't say a word about it. I was given the paperwork and left Station One for the hospital without eating my blood-spattered bagel.

I got another needle in my arm at the hospital, a few stiches, and then I went home. It was a very low chance of getting anything from the little boy and really I could care less. I would do it the same all over again if given the chance.

A week had come and gone since the incident. For some reason everyone was talking about Joey and what happened. It was a good thing right? But why did I still feel so bad? I was working at Station Three on a Friday and was talking to my partner about the run.

He said to me, "Why don't you just call them and find out how he is?"

I said, "I don't want to bother them. They've been through enough without me bothering them."

"Here," he said, handing me the run report. "Here is their phone number on the report." I thought about it, then took the paper.

"Why not?" I said, making my way to the desk in the watch room where the phone was. I hesitated for a minute before finally dialing the number.

"Hello?" said a man's voice.

"Hello. This is Sergeant Johnson from the Fire Department."

"How are you today, Mr. Johnson? How can I help you?" I didn't expect that kind of answer when I called.

"I just wanted to know how Joey is doing." There was a pause for a moment.

"Just a minute," he said. I heard a clunk as he put the phone down. After a long pause, I heard the phone being picked up.

"Hi, Mr. Johnson!" said a tiny voice. "Thanks for saving my life. Bye!" There was another clunk.

"Hello, Mr. Johnson. As you can hear, Joey is doing just fine, and the doctors say he is completely recovered. He was transferred to Children's Hospital the night you rescued him. We thought we would lose him for a while, but he came through with flying colors." He then asked me, "Could we come over to the station and get some pictures with you?"

"Sure," I said. "Anytime." I can't begin to express the relief I felt at that time. The save was complete. Joey and his parents came over for pictures. Joey was running in the apparatus room around the fire trucks like a four year old should. I still have those pictures now.

To top it off, I received a letter of commendation from the Fire Chief, which I have hanging on my office wall. It would have been nice to be able to keep up with the progress of Joey, but I never heard from the family again. I think it's because it was such a traumatic experience that they didn't want to be reminded about how they almost lost their son.

I worked another ten years before my body got too torn up. I retired with thirty years of service on the West Bloom Fire Department. I look back and feel satisfied that I was of service to the com- munity and the families who lived there.

# Retirement Poem

In March of 2009, two officers retired from the West Bloomfield Fire Department. I had worked closely with both of them. To honor the officers, the West Bloomfield Township Supervisor, Michele Economou Ureste wrote the following poem. It is reproduced here with kind permission:

Assistant Fire Chief Ray Riggs (1/1980 – 3/2009)
EMS Captain Mike Flynn (3/1980 – 3/2009)


A career as gratifying and rewarding as this
Is hard to find—you didn't miss
In retirement, however, you will surely miss
Your second family—the one you don't kiss

We worked as a team
Putting our lives on the line
We depended on each other, every time

Assistant fire chief you were four bugles above
What we understood your commitment to us
Your talents span a four-alarm fire
Extending from the percussion to photographer-for-hire
A picture is worth a thousand words
You captured our moments of triumph and fears

EMS captain your bugles sounded our streets
On emergency runs that picked up your feet
Often times it was a "life-and-death" situation
You handled effortlessly with composure and compassion

You have both made a lasting and profound impact here
You touched many lives with skill and with care

We observed, we learned from and we'll think of you
You'll hear the sirens and think of our crew

We'll be in each other's thoughts and prayers
For now and always, throughout the years…

Michele Economou Ureste
West Bloomfield Township Supervisor

# Afterthoughts

I started at West Bloomfield Fire Department on July 1st, 1977. At that time, there were a total of seventeen men employed, and I was number eighteen. There were two paid fire stations; Station One on Orchard Lake Road (fire headquarters) and Station Three on Green Lake Road and Commerce. There were three volunteer stations; Station Two, in the Walnut Lake area, Station Four, in Zox Sub and Station Five on Merlystone off Cooley Lake Road. All three volunteer stations have now been torn down.

We had volunteers until 1984. During the volunteer era, paid firefighters could make volunteer runs on their days off to make extra money. The volunteers and paid men sometimes had issues with each other. One of the old full-time firefighters coined the name for volunteers: "Dicky Liquors." That name was, of course, derogatory at first but after a few years it became the term used for anyone that made volunteer runs. Even the paid men that made volunteer runs called themselves "Dicky Liquors." If we went on a volunteer run on a day off, it was called a "dick run" or a "liquor run" or even a "dick liquor run."

When I started in 1977, there were no paramedics in West Bloomfield Fire Department. In fact, the only two Paramedic Departments in Michigan that I knew of at the time were at Southfield Fire Department and Pontiac Fire Department. I was a basic EMT when I started, but I was in school for my advanced EMT license, which I received the next spring.

The Department got its first paramedic truck in August, 1978. That is the truck I tore the lights off of under the police canopy before we had even used it for a paramedic run. When the first paramedic truck was fixed and we had enough paramedics to run, it was May of 1978. None of us had any experience yet, so we asked Southfield Fire Department to run with us for a month. Paramedic was a brand new field, so there was no place to get experience except on the job. I was one of the first five paramedics on the West Bloomfield Fire Department.

In my first year at WBFD, we had a total of 1,200 runs. When I retired, we had almost seven thousand runs per year. Our first rescue vehicle was dubbed

Life Squad Alpha by Chief Benson and was stationed at Station One. A short time later, we put a second rescue in service, which the Chief named Life Squad Beta. That one was stationed at Station Three. At the time, Station Three was a four to five man station. Each squad was manned by three men. Our squad almost never transported, but instead used a private ambulance for transportation.

I watched Station Four get built in 1978. Life Squad Beta was moved to the new Station Four, along with four to five men. Station Three changed to a two man station. Station One was a six to seven man station. Next, Station Seven was built in 1983. I was stationed there when it opened. Later on, Station Seven was changed to Station Two. Life Squad Delta was put in service there.

The names of Life Squad Alpha, Beta and Delta were changed to Squad One, Two and Seven/Two. Even later, it changed again to Rescue One, Three and Four. Station Seven/Two was a four to five man station and was also made the main station. Station Five was built and opened in December, 2004, three years before I retired. It became the new main station.

West Bloomfield agreed to take over the volunteer Tri-City Fire Department in July, 2003, because the citizens of Orchard Lake, Keego Harbor and Sylvan Lake wanted a full-time fire department.

Some stories I found funny that didn't fit elsewhere in the book are told here. We firefighters had a lot of sayings. One was that someone would ask, "Where is my pen?" Or something like that. This answer would follow, "If it was up your ass, you would know where it's at." One time we went on a tour of the Jewish Community Center. We went on tours of large buildings for fire pre-planning. While on a tour of the very large building, a maintenance worker of German descent was showing us around. He opened most of the doors and showed us what was inside, except for one door which was locked. He couldn't find the key for that room.

We said, "Well, just tell us what is inside the locked room." He answered, with his strong German accent, "Jews."

I asked, "What do you mean, Jews?"

"Ya know, Jews, for the kids." We stood there stunned for a moment until he said, "Jews and crackers." Then we realized he was saying "juice" all along.

Chief Borg, my second Chief, use to refer to the outer stations, like Station Three and Station Four, as "The Outhouses."

"Lonnisms" were quotations from one or our Captains. He would come up to us in the middle of a conversation and say, "I don't know anything about it, but what do you want to know?" He was being serious! The Ten-Code. The first twenty of my thirty years had the Ten-Code for the radio. Station One was 610. Station Seven or Two was 670 or 620. Station Three was 630 and Station Four was 640. Station Five wasn't built during that era. The dispatcher was Station 6. The apparatus at each station was the number of the station it was at.

When the tones went off, the call would go, "Station 6 to 610 you have a run at so and so." The apparatus, like Engine One, would call in when responding, "Engine 1 to station 6. Engine 1 is 10-6 (responding)." Or, "Engine 1 is 10-3 (on the scene)." "Engine 1 is 10-19 (under control). Engine 1 is 10-8 (returning to quarters). Engine1is10-10 (at quarters)."

After about twenty years of my career, the radio talk was changed to clear talk, which is like what I used in the book. We changed from Ten-Code to clear talk and squads to rescues. From non-transport of patients to transporting patients. For the most part I enjoyed the Fire Department, and I wouldn't change a thing.

# Dedication and Acknowledgements

This book is dedicated first to my Savior and Lord, Jesus Christ. In addition, I dedicate this book to my family, including my wife, Wendy, and sons James and Matthew. My mother, Frances, and my father, Edward, who has passed. My father-in-law, Bob Morris, and mother-in-law, Marvis. My sister, Kathy Kobosh, and her husband, Ivan. My brother, Carl. My sister and brother-in-law, Lynn and Jim Poerio.

To the individuals that made up the team of the Fire Department, I thank you all, but especially: West Bloomfield Fire Chief Gregory Flynn, Chief James Poppelreiter, Asst. Chief Raymond Riggs, Captain John Bigger, Lt. Barnard Fante, Lt. Jerome Bismack, Stanley Bridgewater, Robert Jensen, Lt. Thomas Richey, John Steinbach, Martin Kemp, Richard Sprunk, Lt. Harold Burtzloff, Mark Gahan, John Risi, Lt. Michael Flynn, Brian Dalewitz, Captain Michael Watson, Kathy McCormick, Ruth Peterson, and Dora Montgomery.

No on-duty firefighters at West Bloom Fire Department died while I worked there. These are the firefighters I worked with and lost to other causes.

| Name | Status | Date of Death | Notes |
|---|---|---|---|
| James Bowden | | | Died at home |
| Captain Kenneth Barnett | Retired | | Died of cancer that I believe he contracted at a chemical fire. |
| Chief Benson | Retired | | My first Chief |
| Chief Carl Borg | Retired | | My second Chief |
| Leonard Raupp | Retired | | |
| Mike Marsh | Retired | 6-12-14 | |
| Chief/Lt. Roscoe Hunt | Retired | 1-29-11 | |
| Jeff Hiltner | | 2016 | |

Finally I would also like to give a special thanks to those who gave direct support to the book. Wendy for standing by me. Jim Poreo's encouragement helped me get this book finished. Without all the never-ending encouragement and support of my family, this book could not have been written. Wendy and my sister-in-law Lynn on the initial readings of the book.

The last thanks, but not the least, goes to Michele Economou Ureste, West Bloomfield Township Supervisor, who allowed me to make use of her poem.

*G. Stone Johnson*
*October 2016*
*West Bloomfield, Michigan*

# Photographs

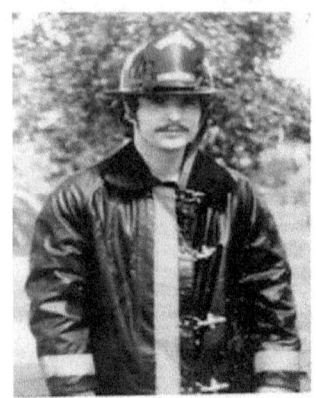

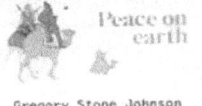

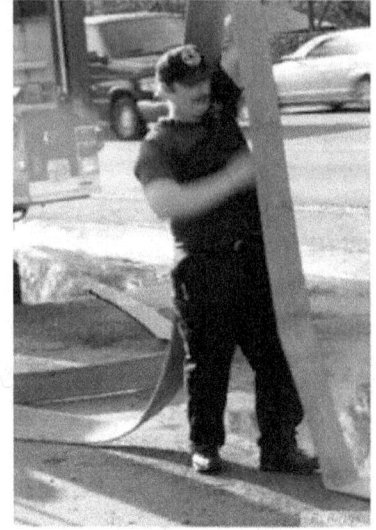

*The author*

*Above: 1977. The early days*

*Above: Emptying a 3 inch hose*

*Below: Next to Rescue One*

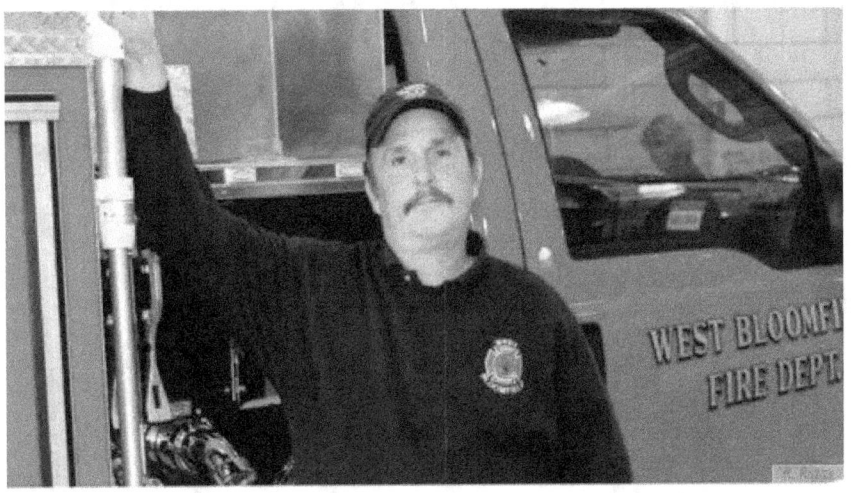

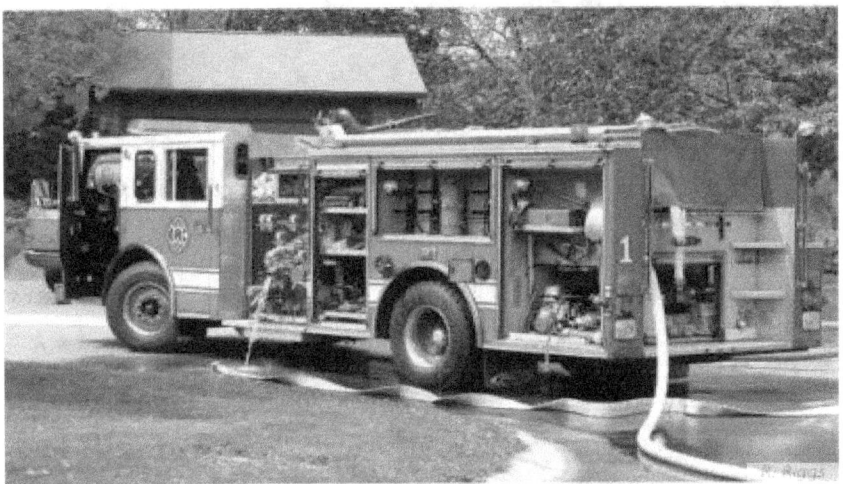

*Engine One at a house fire*

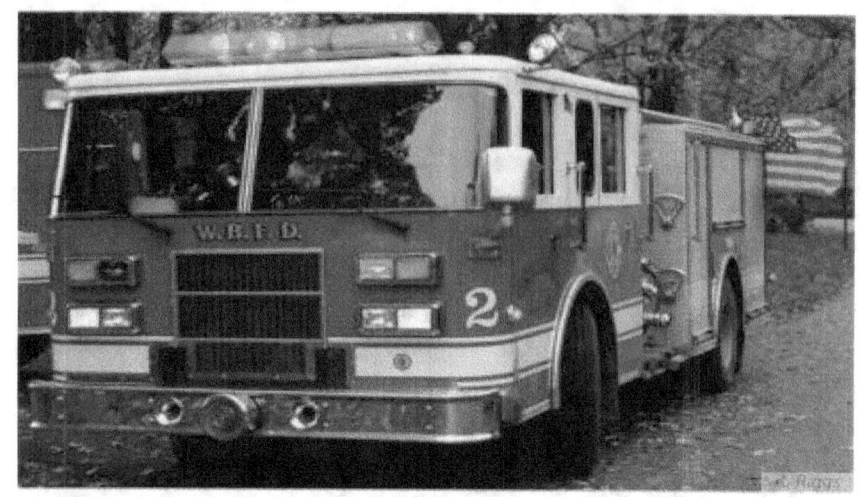
*Engine Two*

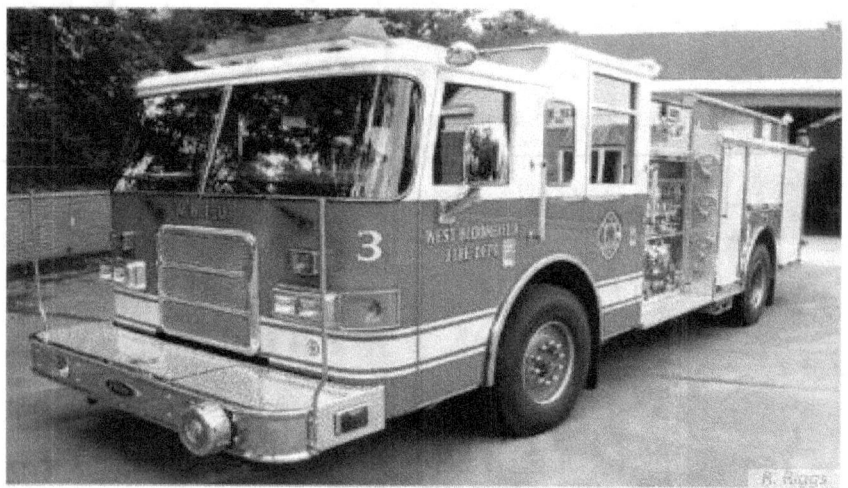
*Engine Three in front of Station Three*

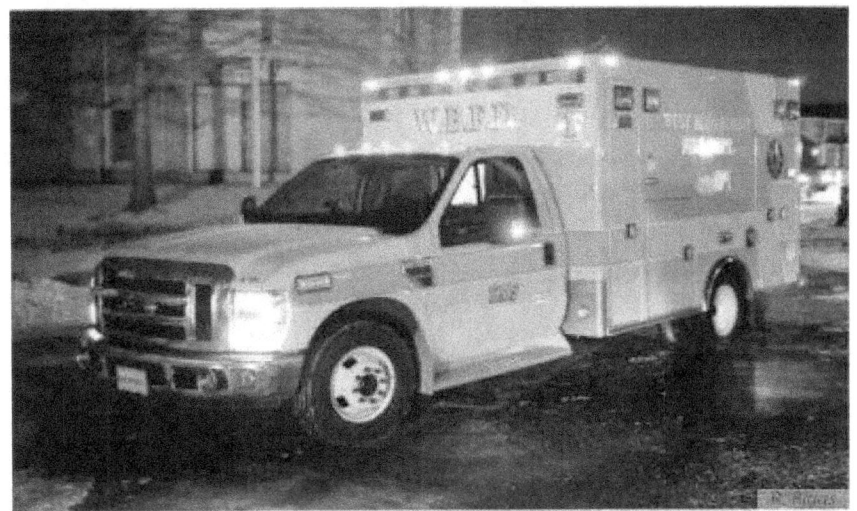
*Rescue One*

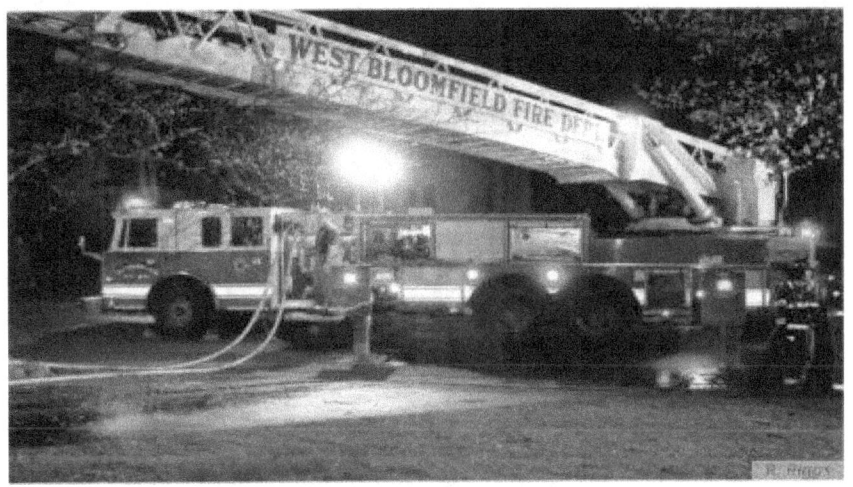
*Ladder One at a structure fire*

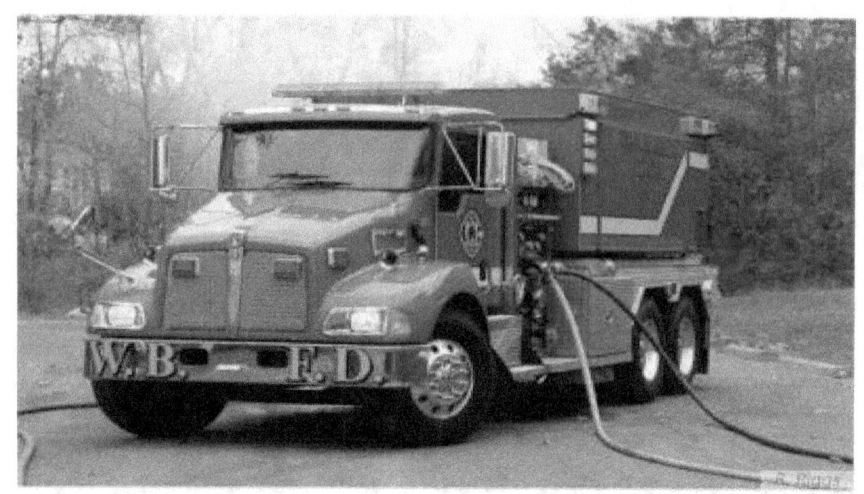

*Tanker Three*

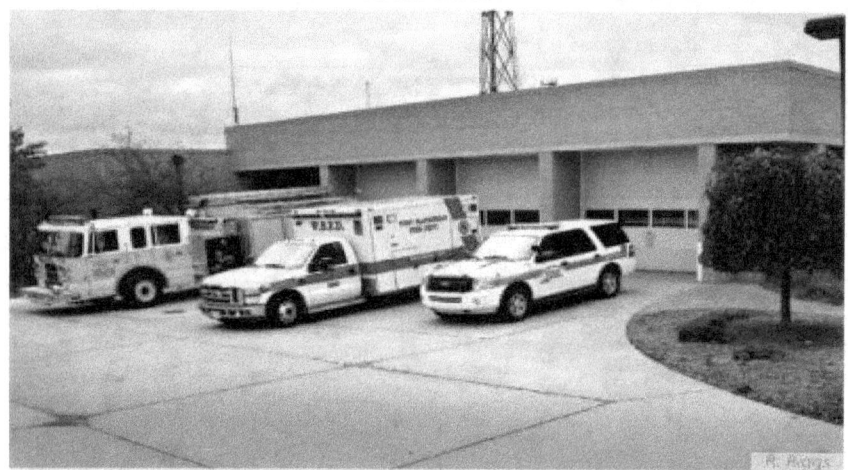

*Station One, Engine One, Rescue One, Cap Car*

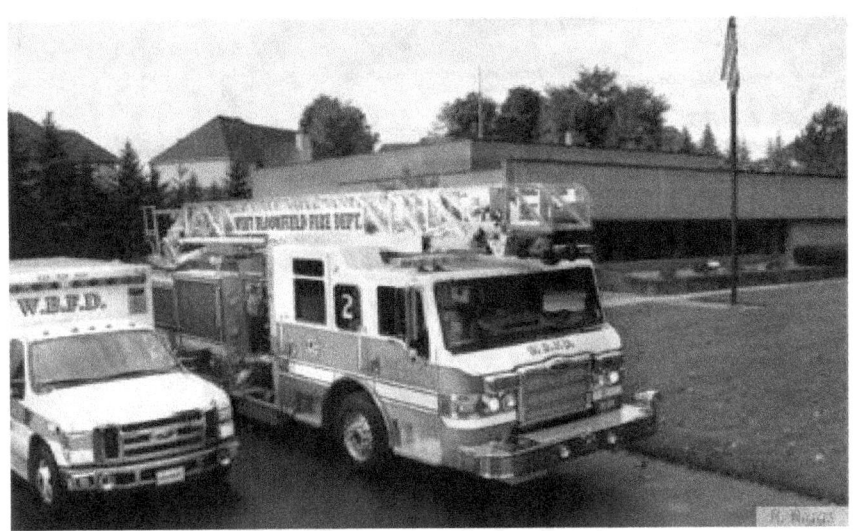

*Station Two, Rescue Two, Ladder Two*

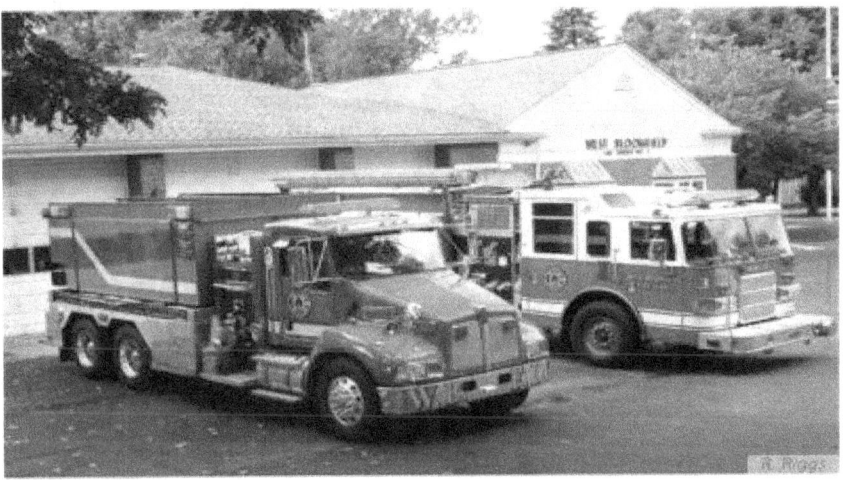

*Station Three, Tanker Three, Engine Three*

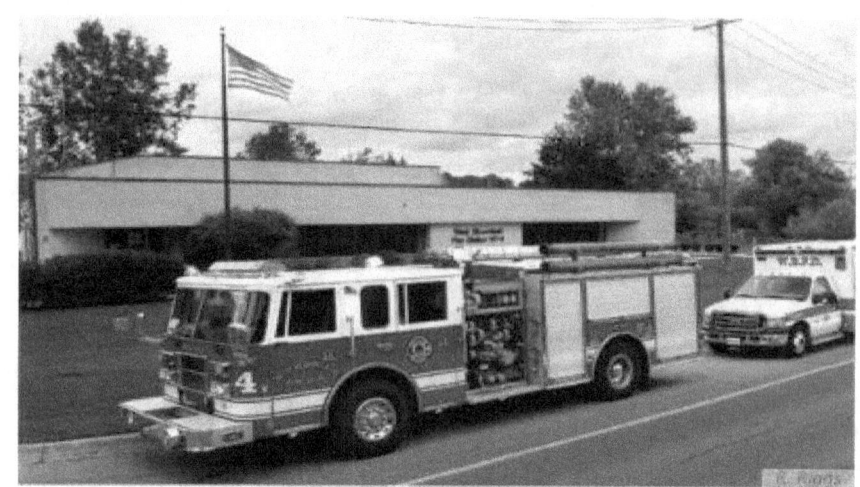
*Station Four, Engine Four, Rescue Four*

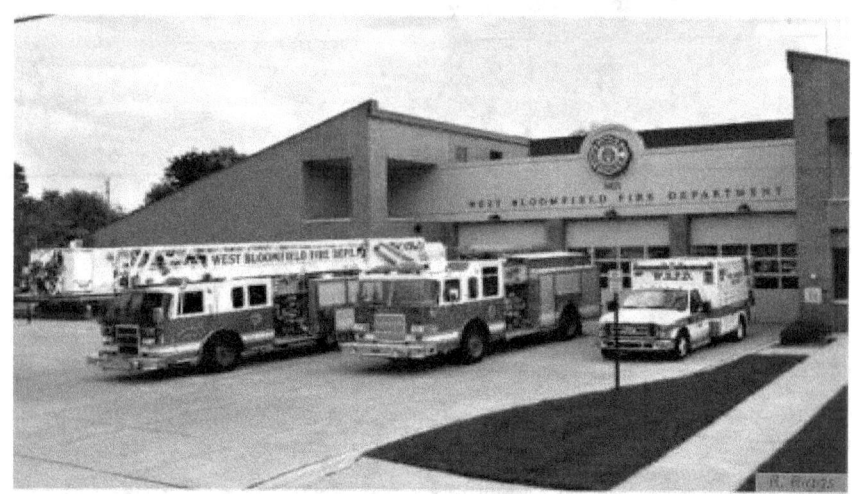
*Station Five, Ladder Five, Engine Five, Rescue Five*

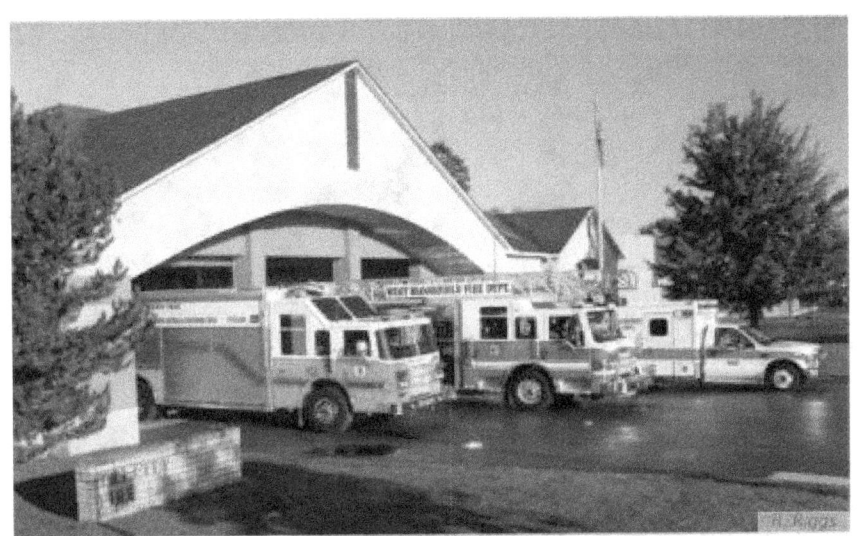
*Station Nine, Hazmat Truck, Ladder Nine, Rescue Nine*

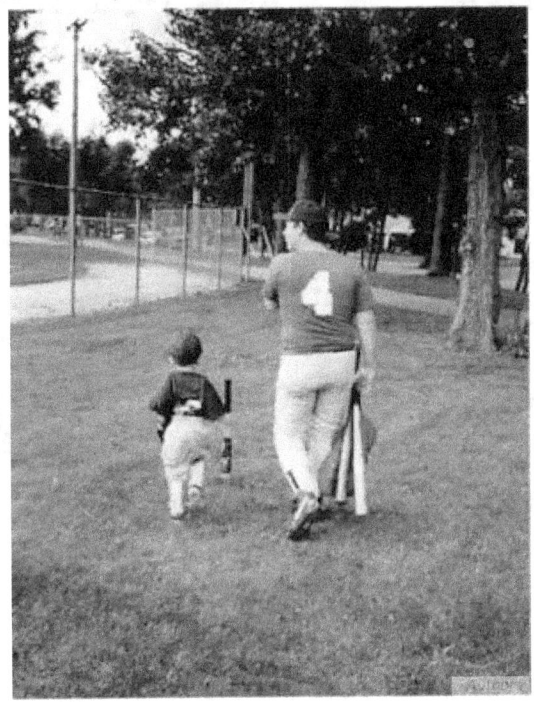
*Above: Softball helper*

*Below: Homecoming greeting. Jimmy on the left, Matt on the right*

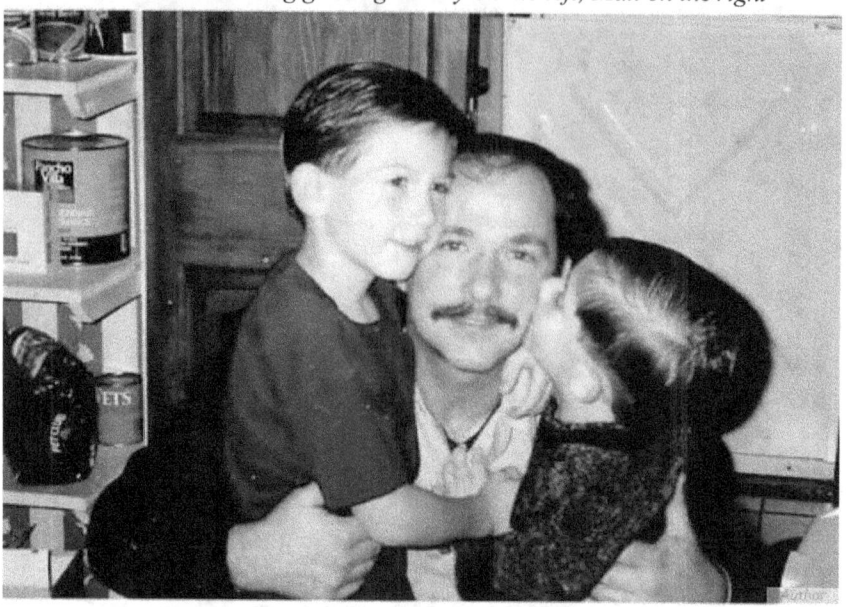

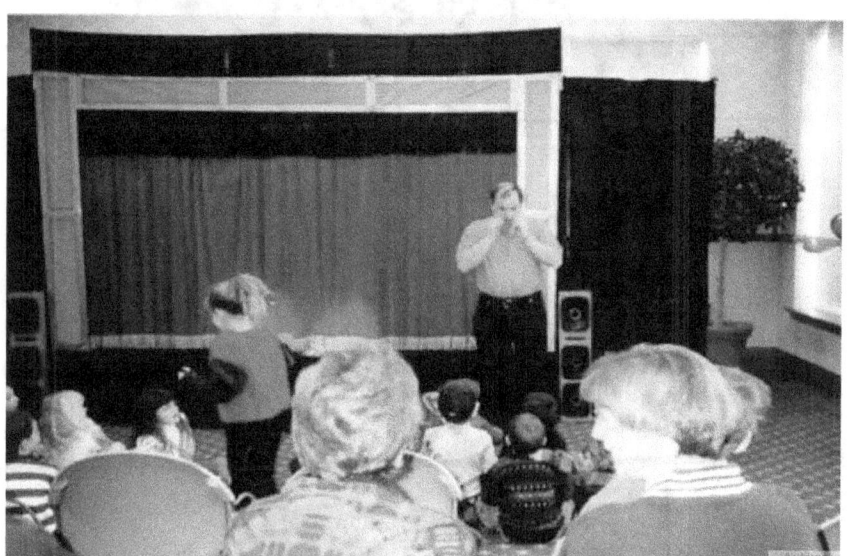

*Above: Marionette show for Christmas party*

*Below: Martial arts, spinning hook kick*

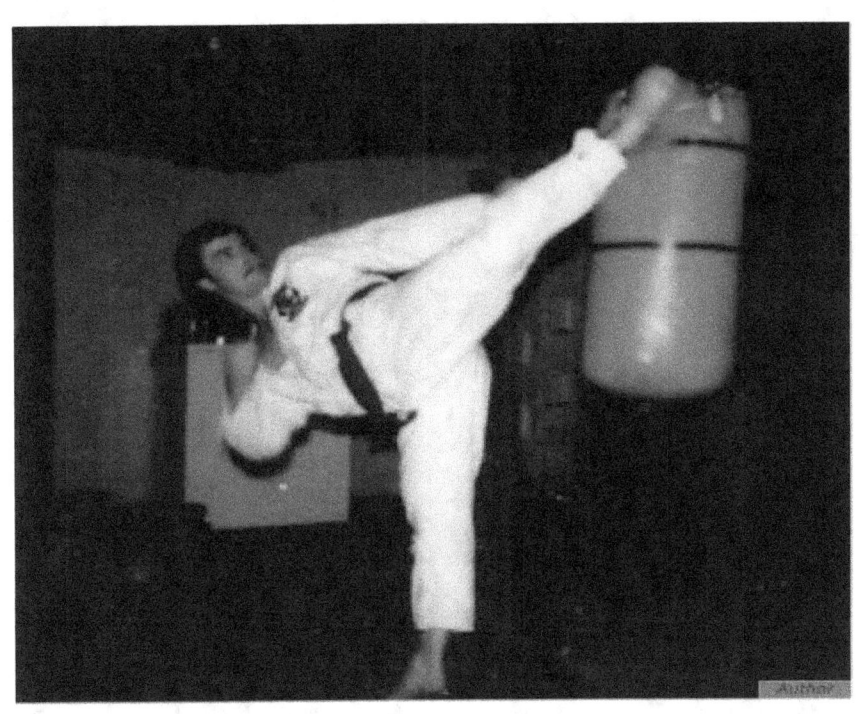

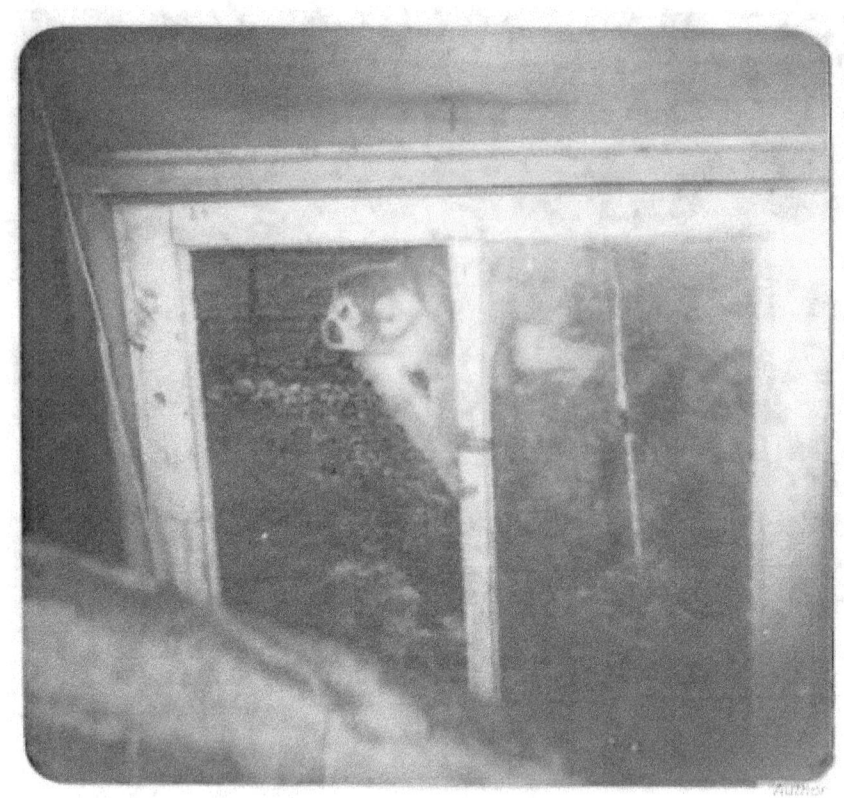
*Beebe the squirrel monkey*

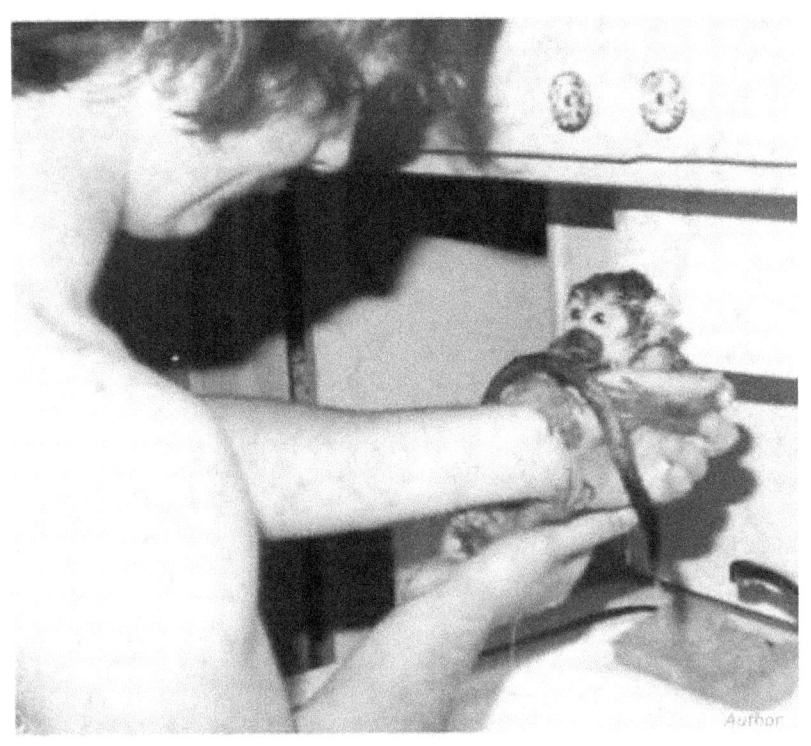

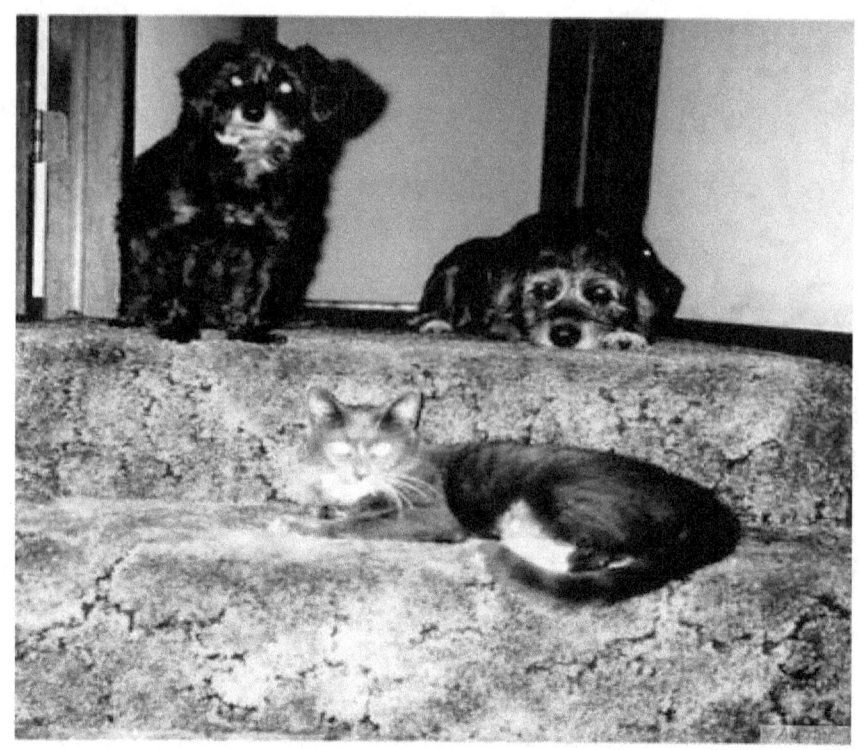

*Above: left, Ninja, right, Mugsy, below, Lassie the cat*

*Below: Mugsy*

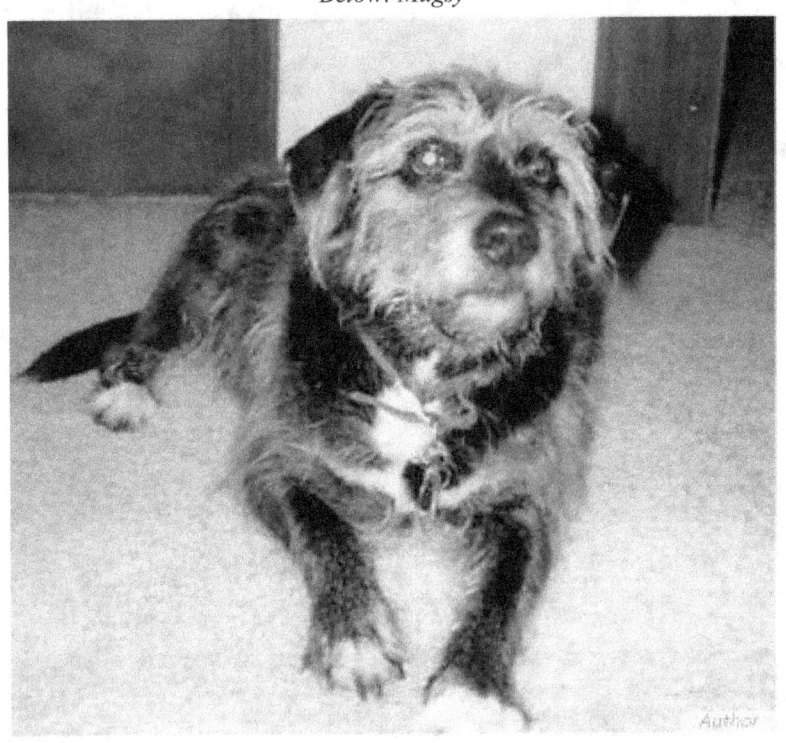

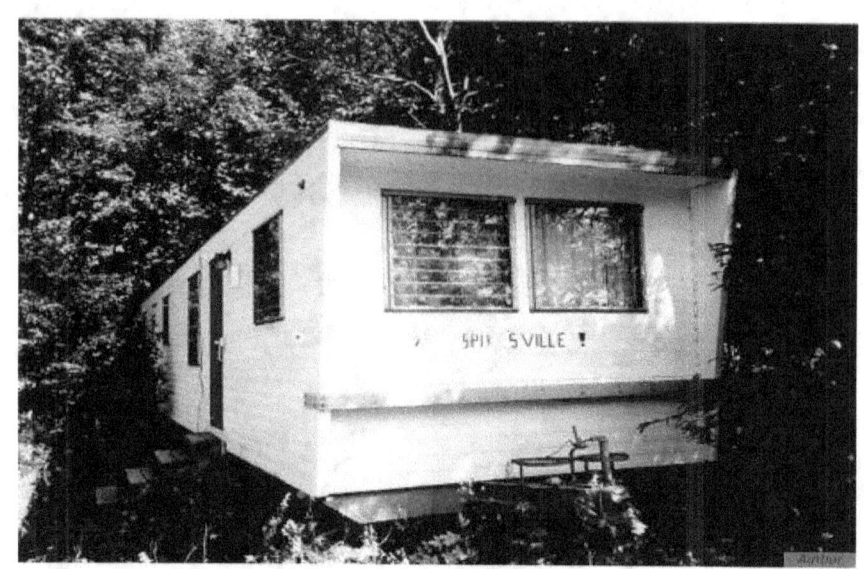

*Above: Up north - the trailer*

*Below: My wound, after falling out of the tree, without stitches*

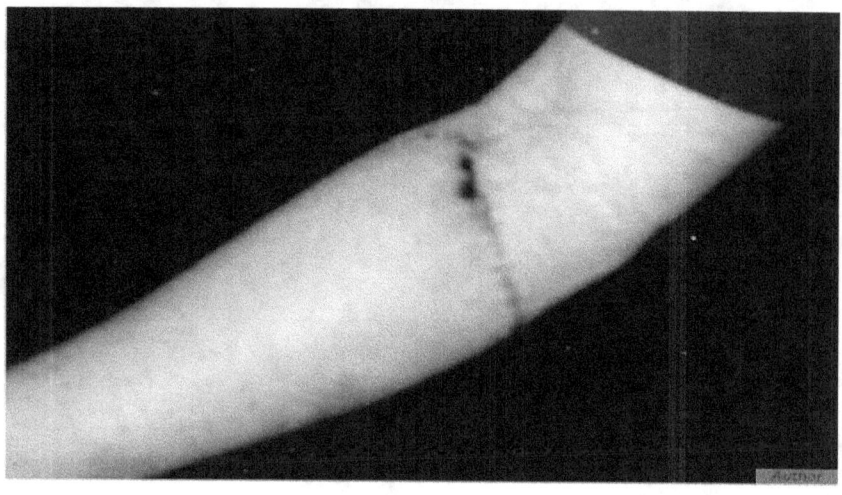

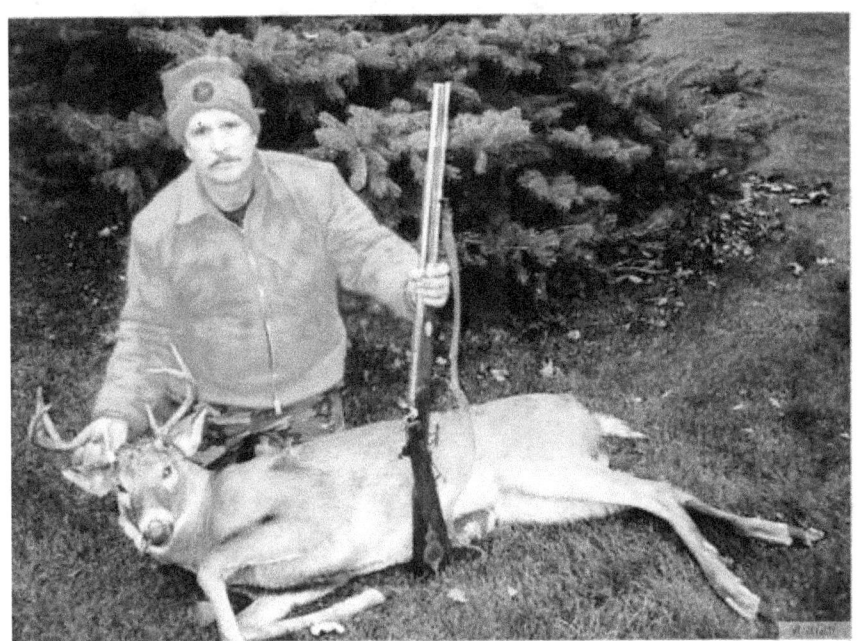

*Deer Hunter with muzzle loader*

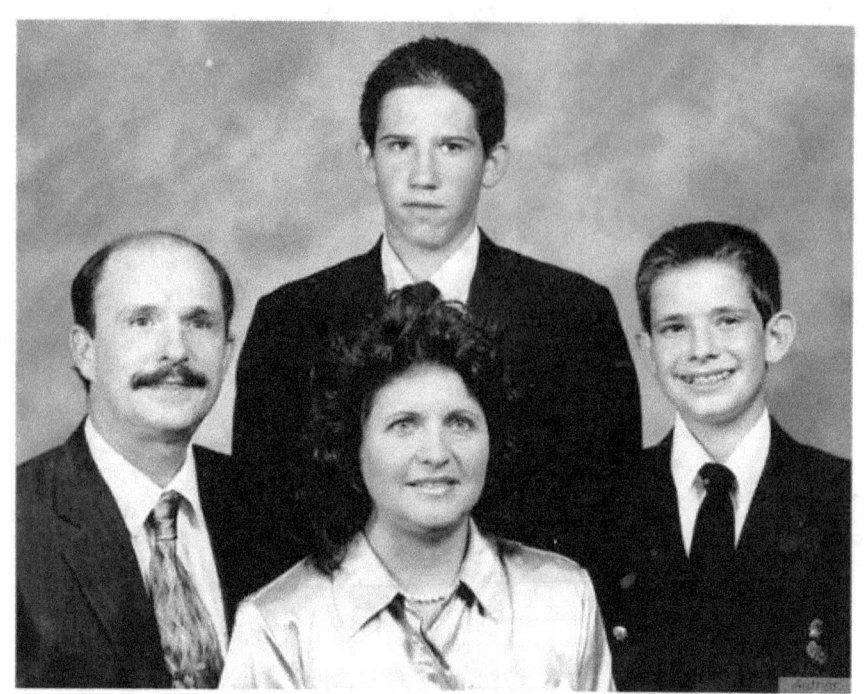
*The Addams Family* ☺

# Glossary

| **Word** | **Definition** |
|---|---|
| agonal respiration | Labored breathing, close to not breathing. Breath comes once in a while. |
| apparatus room | Where the fire fighting and emergency response vehicles are kept. |
| a-systole | No activity of the heart. |
| backboard | A long board used for spinal injuries. |
| Backflash | When the hot gasses in a building get oxygenated. They rapidly catch fire and explode. |
| bag mask | Used for inflating a patient's lungs. Also called the Bag Valve Mask |
| bagging | Forcing the patient to breathe oxygen using a mask connected to a large "bag" that is rhythmically squeezed to cause breathing. |
| bilateral pneumothorax | A condition where there is air around the lungs. With- out treatment, the lungs will collapse. |
| blood pressure | A measure of the pressure of the blood in the arteries between heart beats: normal is 120/80 |
| BPM | Beats per minute; a unit to measure the heart beat rate- normal ranges from 72-80 to 100. |
| bunker pants | Fire gear you wear like pants to protect the lower body. |
| butt the ladder | One or two firefighters anchor the ladder, giving the climbing firefighters a more stable climb. |
| cervical collar | A medical device used to support the neck of a patient to prevent further injury. |
| CPR | Cardiopulmonary Resuscitation |
| Cricoid process | The cartilage covering the vocal chords. |
| cross lays | Refers to the way the 1-1/2 inch hose is laid out on top of the apparatus for quick fire attack. |
| Defibrillate | Applying an electric shock to restart the heart. |
| depressed skull fracture | A skull fracture where the bone is pushed into the brain. |
| dextrose and water | A sugar and water IV solution. |

| | |
|---|---|
| Dispatcher | Located at the police station, this person receives all calls and sends police and fire department rescues to the address of the emergency. |
| donkey dicks | What the firefighters called sausages. |
| dopamine | A drug used to make the blood pressure go up. |
| double clutch | A transmission type, where the clutch is engaged twice to change gears. |
| E.C.G. | Electrocardiogram-a diagnostic tool used to assess the function of the heart. |
| e.t.o.h. | Referring to someone who has been drinking alcohol. |
| Endotracheal tube | A tube inserted via the patient's mouth into the trachea. |
| Epiglottis | The flap of flesh that covers the airway when a person swallows. |
| Epinephrine | Also known as adrenaline, it is used to stimulate the heart. It is also used to treat severe allergic reactions. |
| fire turnout gear | The gear worn by firefighters when attacking a fire: fire coat, helmet, boots, bunker pants. |
| flat line | The monitor of heart electrical activity goes flat, indicates the patient has died. |
| fog nozzle | Produces a fog spray from a fire hose. |
| Gomer run | A non-emergency run; for example to a residence of an older person who needs non-life threatening assistance. |
| governor | A device used to control the speed of a machine. |
| hose reel | Located on the back or side of Engine. One inch hose is 100 feet of one inch rubber hose used for small fires. |
| inferior vein cava | Major artery coming out of the heart and going down through the abdomen. |
| Intracardiac syringe | Used to give injections of medicines directly into the heart chambers for fast effect. |
| Intubate | Refers to the insertion of a breathing tube into the trachea to assist with manual respiration. |
| IV | Mostly refers to a catheter (tube) inserted into a vein for administration of IV fluids or medicines. |
| jaws of life | Hydraulic-powered rescue tools; used when the patient is trapped inside a vehicle. |

| | |
|---|---|
| Joules | A measure of electrical energy. |
| K | Shorthand over the radio for "killed." |
| Kelly days | The middle day off of the three days off. |
| Laryngoscope | A medical instrument, in the shape of an "L," with a light on the end; used to intubate a patient. |
| larynx | The vocal chords. |
| LIFEPAK 10 | Brand of a portable heart monitor and defibrillator. |
| ME | Medical Examiners are medically qualified officers who pick up dead bodies from sites. |
| mg | Milligrams; a small unit of measurement. |
| normal sinus rhythm | Normal electrical rhythm. |
| OFU | Other F-ing Unit. |
| Open fracture | Broken bone that breaks through the skin. |
| p.t.o. | Lever used to connect the Engine to other apparatus. |
| PIA | Personal Injury Accident; involving a person and a vehicle. |
| Rescue | A heavy vehicle containing apparatus used in medical and rescue situations. |
| Ringer's lactate solution | A saline solution used for trauma. A blood expander. |
| Silvadene | Silver sulfadiazine; a medical ointment used to treat burns. |
| stokes basket | A litter used to move a patient from a hazardous position and challenging terrain. |
| subby | A rookie in the department. |
| through and through injury | A gunshot wound where the bullet entered and exited the body. |
| trachea | The windpipe, which connects the larynx and the lungs. |
| Traction | A mechanical pull; used to treat a fractured limb to correct alignment or relieve pressure. |
| variable stream nozzle | A nozzle that allows the firefighter to change the pow- er/force of the stream of water without taking time to change nozzles; from fog to straight stream. |
| ventricular-tachycardia | A condition where the heart goes into cardiac arrest. Usually there is no pulse. |

| | |
|---|---|
| v-fib | Ventricular fibrillation is a serious cardiac rhythmic disturbance where the lower chambers can no longer pump blood. Full arrest. |
| volunteer/paid on call position. | Part-time or used as-needed, rather than a full-time |
| wireman | Gets to work at the last minute |